DELIVERING PERSO
HEALTH BUDGET

A guide to policy and practice

Vidhya Alakeson

First published in Great Britain in 2014 by

Policy Press
University of Bristol
6th Floor
Howard House
Queen's Avenue
Clifton
Bristol BS8 1SD
UK
Tel +44 (0)117 331 5020
Fax +44 (0)117 331 5367
e-mail pp-info@bristol.ac.uk
www.policypress.co.uk

North American office:
Policy Press
c/o The University of Chicago Press
1427 East 60th Street
Chicago, IL 60637, USA
t: +1 773 702 7700
f: +1 773-702-9756
e:sales@press.uchicago.edu
www.press.uchicago.edu

© Policy Press 2014

British Library Cataloguing in Publication Data
A catalogue record for this book is available from the British Library

Library of Congress Cataloging-in-Publication Data
A catalog record for this book has been requested

ISBN 978 1 44730 852 2 paperback
ISBN 978 1 44730 853 9 hardcover

The right of Vidhya Alakeson to be identified as author of this work has been asserted by her in accordance with the 1988 Copyright, Designs and Patents Act.

Cover design by Qube Design Associates, Bristol
Printed and bound in Great Britain by CPI Group (UK) Ltd, Croydon, CR0 4YY
The Policy Press uses environmentally responsible print partners

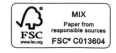

Contents

List of tables and figures

Tables

Figures

Acknowledgements

I would like to thank all those whose stories and experiences of having a personal health budget have illuminated this book. Yours is the most powerful evidence that this approach works. I would also like to thank all the pilot sites with whom I have had the opportunity to work and from whom I have learnt about the challenges of implementing even the best idea.

I am hugely grateful to so many individuals with whom I have worked on personal health budgets and self-direction over the last seven years and from whom I have learnt so much, including: Alison Austin, Carey Bamber, Rita Brewis, Pamela Doty, Dick Dougherty, Simon Duffy, Jo Fitzgerald, Jon Glasby, Kevin Lewis, Kevin Mahoney, Tricia Nicoll, Rachel Perkins, Zoe Porter, Martin Routledge, Gill Ruecroft, Gill Stewart, Julie Stansfield, Shawn Terrell and Pam Werner. You span both sides of the Atlantic but are joined by a belief in the expertise of individuals to improve their own lives, given half a chance. Some of you commented on drafts of the book for which a special thank you, and to Rob, thank you for making pictures of my words. I am also very grateful to Ali Shaw at Policy Press for guiding this book from idea to reality.

Prologue

Stephen's story

In 2008, Stephen had an accident and sustained a spinal injury which left him tetraplegic and completely paralysed from the shoulders down. After three months in intensive care and a further eight months at a rehabilitation unit in Sheffield, Stephen returned home in August 2009. The period following Stephen's return home was his darkest. In rehab, the entire focus was on what Stephen could do and his partner, Nicola, was trained in the specialist care he needed. Stephen and Nicola were supported to learn what was necessary to be able to live a full and active life in the future. Everything changed when they returned home.

They chose a larger care agency because they were assured it would be better able to cope with Stephen's needs, but according to Nicola, it was 'hell on earth'. There were early warning signs that things would not work out. Instead of covering all his needs, Stephen's care plan only focused on the physical side and did not say anything about Stephen as a father, partner or other parts of his life. Before Stephen's accident he renovated houses and was a part-time househusband, but there was no mention of the support he might need to continue his interests or simple fatherly tasks such as school runs, mealtimes, bath times and bedtimes. Agency staff were instructed not to do menial tasks considered social care such as emptying bins or changing a light bulb, even though their role was to support Stephen to be an active family member.

Stephen was getting more and more depressed, and Nicola was getting more stressed because she was also working full time. Stephen felt that they were not getting value for money. The agency's recruitment process was not personalised; there was nothing about Stephen in the process with which staff could connect. The agency would often send carers who couldn't drive, which meant that Stephen couldn't get out and about. In his first autumn and winter at home, Stephen did not leave the lounge for up to three weeks at a time. He rarely asked for care or support because he didn't relate to the care team and didn't want them in his house. While the agency ticked every box as far as the Care Quality Commission was concerned, no one ever asked Stephen's opinion about his care. No one took him seriously as a customer, and purely from a health point of view,

Stephen had three chest infections in his first three months at home because he wasn't getting the passive exercises he needed and was stuck in the lounge not getting any fresh air.

Fortunately, Stephen had a review after three months when it became clear that he could become part of the Nottinghamshire Primary Care Trust personal health budget pilot. Stephen's personal health budget was a year in the planning. The focus of his plan was to find a purpose and a meaning in his new life and to ensure that Stephen could be actively involved with his children again. The children had found the accident very hard and had stopped spending time in the house. It was important to Stephen and Nicola to create a situation that was comfortable for them.

With his personal health budget, Stephen has hired his own team of dedicated carers. He doesn't look to employ people who have care experience. He prefers to train staff to accommodate his own specific needs and looks for people who respect the fact that he is in control and who are willing to listen and take direction. Stephen decides who works, and when, based on his plans for the week. The carers also feel part of a team and can help each other by covering holidays.

Stephen provides comprehensive professional training for all his team, but this is only completed when Stephen is comfortable with their level of competence. The agency would often send untrained carers who did not have the skills and confidence to meet Stephen's needs. For example, he cannot cough and needs to be assisted to cough. On one occasion, the agency sent a young woman with only six months' experience of generalist care who did not know Stephen well enough to care for him alone overnight. At the same time, when Stephen's care coordinator realised that the family was going out for lunch without a carer, she considered it a safeguarding issue that put Stephen at risk, despite the fact Nicola is fully trained and more knowledgeable about Stephen's care than anyone else.

Nicola feels that they would not have been able to manage a personal health budget when Stephen first came home. She feels that it helps to have a care package in place for the first six to eight months and that you can use that time to put your own personalised package in place. She says running a personal health budget for a large package is a lot of work; you have to go into it with your eyes wide open. However, there are real advantages. Although the amount of money available for Stephen's care is the same as before, Stephen is able to convert this into more variable and flexible hours of support than he could with an agency. This has enabled him to hire two gardeners and to get back outside. He can direct them and it gives him something he can do with his youngest daughter. This means that Stephen can be a dad without Nicola always having to be around because he needs two-to-one support when he is in charge of his very young daughter.

Stephen has also used his personal health budget to buy an iPad and a bracket for his wheelchair so he can browse easily. This allows him to use the internet and shop and, most importantly, to read a bedtime story to his daughter. He has also bought an iMac with voice-activated software. The iMac is fast enough for the voice activation to work quickly and smoothly and this means that Stephen can do simple things like reading a newspaper with relative ease. He has also bought a specialist hoist, which allows him to be hoisted into his classic convertible car, which he is now able to enjoy once again. Finally, Stephen has used some of his personal health budget to buy a powered 4x4 wheelchair that enables him to have a more active outdoor lifestyle than his original wheelchair allowed. In the new wheelchair, he can be on the beach with his young daughter or go across muddy footpaths on country walks.

Stephen and Nicola are so passionate about self-directed support for people with long-term health conditions and disabilities that they are using their lived experience of personal health budgets and Nicola's extensive experience in recruitment and human resources to run their own personal health budget agency, Solo Support Services. They offer a 'third party' arrangement for people who don't want or are not able to have a direct payment.

Source: Stephen's story is based on the author's interview with Nicola Darby, December 2012, and reviewed by Stephen in February 2013.

Introduction

In 2001, the prestigious Institute of Medicine published a groundbreaking report that defined the six dimensions of healthcare quality. Alongside more predictable dimensions such as efficiency, effectiveness and safety was patient-centredness (Institute of Medicine, 2011). More than a decade on and we need little reminder of how often care in the National Health Service (NHS) fails to deliver on this dimension of quality. From the inhumane treatment of some of the most vulnerable members of our society at Winterbourne View Hospital (DH, 2012a) and the levels of neglect revealed by the inquiry into deaths at Stafford Hospital (Francis, 2013) to repeated concerns about the lack of dignity afforded older people in hospital (CQC, 2011), our record on patient-centredness is patchy at best. Addressing the International Forum on Quality and Safety in Healthcare, Dr Don Berwick, one of the foremost experts on healthcare quality improvement, described his fear of becoming a patient and the loss of dignity and control that entails:

> It scares me to be made helpless before my time, to be made ignorant when I want to know, to be made to sit when I want to stand or to be alone when I need to hold my wife's hand or to eat when I do not wish to eat or to be named when I do not wish to be named or to be told when I wish to be asked or to be awoken when I wish to sleep. You can call it patient-centredness if you choose. But I suggest to you that this is the core. It is the property of care that welcomes me to assert my humanity and my individuality and my uniqueness. And if we be healers, I suggest to you that this is not the route to the point, it is the point. (Berwick, 2009a)

Berwick's comments on the centrality of patient-centredness are viewed as those of a radical. It is a strange feature of public services, including the NHS, that the notion that services are designed for and respond to their users is considered radical. The same idea would be mundane in other industries where providers survive by virtue of their ability to respond to customers. Of course, public services are not simple commodities, but there is no shortage of evidence of services run without due consideration of the needs and preferences of those who use them. Take the care agency that can only arrive to get someone up two hours after that person needs to be at work or the group home that only serves its residents a cold drink unless they fill in a form to 'apply' for a hot one. Worse still, as Berwick describes, is the loss of agency and dignity that all too often accompanies stepping into the service user role. Your opinion suddenly counts for less. Your expertise remains untapped and you are forced to fit into a service that was designed for someone like you, but not for you.

In *Development as Freedom* (1999), Nobel Laureate Amartya Sen sets out a powerful argument that the way public services achieve their outcomes matters as well as the outcomes themselves. People value a process in which they are involved more than one in which they are not involved, even if the outcome is identical. The value of public services should be measured not only in the improvements they make to employment or educational attainment but in the possibilities they create for individuals to exercise their own choices and to pursue their own priorities. In healthcare, the emphasis on scientific evidence creates a focus on improving people's clinical functioning without equal consideration of how the necessary interventions affect their quality of life, wellbeing and sense of control over their own lives. These things are secondary when they should be at the centre of how we judge the NHS, as Berwick argues. What is the value of evidence-based care if, in managing a person's symptoms, medication erodes that person's ability to do the things that matter most to them?

Personal health budgets (PHBs) are a radical new tool to create an NHS that genuinely responds to the needs, preferences and priorities of the people who use it – a truly patient-centred NHS that empowers patients to define their own objectives and shape their own care. They are one example of the 'personalisation' of public services that is seeking to improve outcomes for people by giving them greater choice and control, recognising that a sense of agency itself is a powerful tool to change lives. The move to give individuals greater control in public services is not unique to the UK. It is an international trend, transforming services in health, social care, education and welfare from continental Europe and the US to Australia.

PHBs alter the balance of power in the NHS to put the expertise that individuals and their families bring to the care of long-term conditions and disabilities on an equal footing with the scientific knowledge and clinical experience of professionals. Through an individualised care planning process, they allow budget holders to define the health and wellbeing outcomes they want to achieve and how those outcomes are best met. For example, the best thing to improve a child's asthma may be double-glazing to reduce damp in the house and the best form of pain relief for a person with multiple sclerosis may be a weekly massage.

Access to these alternative solutions is possible with a PHB because critically, the individual controls the financial resources that the NHS would previously have spent on their behalf. Clinical expertise remains important in this context, but it is at the service of individuals, to be drawn on when required – 'on tap rather than on top' (Repper and Perkins, 2003, p 27).

In 2009, the Department of Health began a three-year pilot of PHBs involving 64 commissioning organisations (at the time, primary care trusts, PCTs) and covering a range of long-term conditions, including chronic obstructive pulmonary disease (COPD), diabetes, long-term neurological conditions, mental health and stroke, as well as individuals receiving NHS continuing healthcare (CHC), maternity services and end of life care. Of the 64 sites, 20 were involved in an in-depth evaluation that compared the outcomes and experiences of 1,000 people using a PHB to manage their care with those of 1,000 people receiving NHS care as usual. The evaluation demonstrated that PHBs improve the lives of people with long-term conditions and disabilities. They are a cost-effective way to improve quality of life and wellbeing and their impact is greater the more they offer genuine choice and control to individuals. Confirming the central importance of agency, the final evaluation report recognises that much of the improvement for PHB holders stems from the choice and control intrinsic to the approach (Forder et al, 2012).

In its first mandate for the NHS in England, the government calls for the NHS to become 'dramatically better at involving patients and their carers, and empowering them to manage and make decisions about their own care and treatment' (DH, 2012b, p 9). As part of fulfilling this objective and based on the success of the pilots, the government confirmed in November 2012 that PHBs will become an established feature of the NHS, starting with the 56,000 people with highly complex, long-term health needs who receive CHC (DH, 2012c). As of April 2014, everyone eligible for CHC will have the right to ask for their care to be delivered as a PHB and the NHS will have to be in a position to respond. The right will also cover children with special educational needs and disabilities who will be able to have an integrated budget across the NHS, social care and education. As of 2015, commissioners should be ready to offer a PHB to anyone with a long-term condition who could benefit from one. The legislation needed to support the national roll-out of PHBs is expected to be in place by autumn 2013 (DH, 2013).

While PHBs have a philosophical connection to other shared decision-making initiatives introduced into the NHS in the last decade, such as the Year of Care (2011) and the Expert Patient Programme (Rogers et al, 2006), they nevertheless represent an enormous culture change for the service. PHBs require an entirely new orientation towards individuals who require care: they are experts with assets rather than a set of diagnoses and deficits. For clinical professionals, seeing their relationship with their patients as a partnership between two experts with different sets of knowledge is to unlearn much of what they have been trained to do. PHBs also demand a different provider market, more closely shaped by the views of individuals and families, with greater diversity of providers, a different service mix and more responsiveness from traditional NHS providers. This changes the role not only of providers but also of commissioners at a time when the NHS is under enormous financial pressure simply to keep up with the pace of demographic and technological change. However, as this book sets out to demonstrate, these are not insurmountable challenges and the rewards are great.

This book is the culmination of seven years of personal experience working to develop and deliver the concept of PHBs in the UK and US. From 2010 to 2013, I worked closely with sites involved in the PHB pilot programme, helping them to figure out how to implement PHBs to get the best results for individuals. As a consequence, the advice and examples you will find in this book are drawn from practice, not theory, and from a sound understanding of the challenges of making change happen in a complex healthcare system like the NHS. Over the last three years I have also had the privilege of interviewing and getting to know several PHB holders and their families. Some of their stories and experiences are included in the book. They are the best evidence that this approach can work and change people's lives for the better.

The book has two purposes. The first is to make the case for PHBs as a new way of delivering healthcare that has already made a positive difference to hundreds of people's lives and that has the potential to transform care for thousands more. PHBs present an opportunity to preserve the fundamental principles of the NHS and also to broaden its focus from delivering healthcare to supporting people with health needs to live their lives to the fullest extent possible. This comes at a time when the need for cost-effective approaches to the management of long-term conditions has never been more pressing. Long-term conditions already account for the majority of spending in the NHS and, with an ageing population, the cost can only rise (Alakeson and Rosen, 2011).

The book's second purpose is to serve as a guide for academics, policymakers, managers and practitioners in the NHS, whether you are simply curious about PHBs or actively involved in their implementation. The book can be read from start to finish and will give you a complete overview of what PHBs are, what they are for and what needs to happen to support their implementation. However, you can also treat the book more as a reference manual and consult different chapters for an overview of specific issues.

Section 1 starts with an overview of personalisation across public services. In doing so, it puts developments in the NHS within the broader context of public service reform. It then goes on to introduce PHBs and their purpose. It traces the roots of PHBs back to the independent living movement of the 1970s and 1980s, discusses their connection to other initiatives in the NHS for the management of long-term conditions and assesses the strength of the evidence base, drawing on studies from the UK and internationally.

Section 2 focuses on the steps required to implement PHBs. After an overview of the entire process, one chapter is devoted to each of the main types of infrastructure required for PHBs: a system for allocating resources to individuals; a system to provide support to budget holders, including around care planning; and options for how the money in a PHB can be held and managed.

Section 3 puts PHBs into a wider NHS context. It looks at where they fit within the government's programme of reform as set out in the 2012 Health and Social Care Act. It goes on to set out the implications of PHBs for commissioners, clinical professionals and providers. In each case, it presents strategies for how necessary changes can be introduced, transitions managed and challenges overcome. Finally, the Conclusion highlights possibilities for the future direction of personalisation.

A note on terminology

There is a complex muddle of terms used internationally to describe an approach to service delivery that gives choice and control to individuals. For the purposes of this book, the following terms are used:

- *Personalisation* is used in a UK context to describe the concept of giving choice and control to individuals across public services. When referring to the same concept internationally, the term *self-direction* is used.
- When referring in general to the allocation of resources to individuals, the book uses the term *individual budget*. The term *personal health budget* is only used in the context of the NHS, and

personal budget is used in the context of UK social care as that is the commonly used term in that field.

Section I

Introducing personal health budgets

ONE

Personalisation across public services

The purpose of this book is to set out the objectives underpinning the roll-out of personal health budgets in the National Health Service (NHS); to provide an overview of how PHBs can be implemented to best deliver on those objectives; and to identify some of the barriers to implementation and how they can be overcome. Within the NHS, PHBs are highly innovative and present new challenges to commissioners, clinicians and individuals. But just as they have a shared history with personal budgets in social care (discussed in Chapter 3), they are also part of a set of new initiatives that are driving personalisation across public services. At the heart of each initiative is a common set of principles, a similar design and a common delivery mechanism – an individual budget and a personalised plan for how the individual budget can best be deployed to help people achieve their goals. This chapter puts PHBs in the NHS into their wider context and looks at the spread of personalisation across public services.

The principles underpinning personalisation across public services

- A new relationship between the citizen and the state based on co-production.
- Self-determination expressed through informed choice, control and accountability for the individual – do less *to* people and more *with* them.
- Government should step back, making space for individuals to lead their lives as they choose.
- A more preventative approach with support provided in a timely way.
- The ability for individuals to use resources in new ways.
- Making full use of the expertise of the voluntary and private sectors, disabled people's organisations and peer support.
- Affordable and sustainable support, with transition costs grounded in austerity measures.
- Local freedom and accountability, with Whitehall as adviser.

Source: Adapted from an Office for Disability Issues workshop facilitated by the author, August 2011

From personalisation to open public services

As discussed later in Chapter 3, the concept of personalisation arose out of a complex interaction between the disabled people's movement for independent living and the work of think tanks and policymakers. By 2007, it had become a central idea within public service reform under the then Labour government and the governing idea in adult social care. Personalisation provided a softer alternative to market-based reforms in health and education that sought to extend choice through competition. The basic concept that services should be tailored to the needs of those who use them is one with which it is hard to disagree.

In fact, the ongoing popularity of the concept of personalisation owes much to its capaciousness. It is loose enough to receive support from across the political spectrum, with each party lending it its own particular emphasis (Needham, 2011). For Labour, it is a route to greater individual empowerment and a way to shift the relationship between the individual and the state from one in which the state does things *for* people to one in which it does things *with* people (Mulgan, 2012). For Liberals, it is an approach to public services that puts power in the hands of people to decide which goals to pursue to improve their lives (Reeves, 2010). When announcing the roll-out of PHBs in November 2012, Liberal Democrat Health Minister, Norman Lamb MP, described them as a 'liberal' approach to NHS reform. For those on the right, personalisation can be seen to emphasise personal responsibility and market-based solutions that exploit consumer power rather than state-led action. As such, personalisation is a term well suited to Coalition politics as it provides room for different definitions to coexist.

The current Coalition government built on the foundations laid by Labour through the publication of its *Open public services* White Paper in July 2011 (HM Government, 2011). At the heart of its framework for public services set out in the White Paper are choice and decentralisation: the government should increase choice wherever possible, and services should be devolved to the lowest possible level. In the case of policing, this may be devolution from national to local government and for leisure services, from local government to communities themselves. In the case of services such as health, education and housing support that are used on an individual basis, the White Paper commits to put power in the hands of people. This transfer of power, the White Paper argues, is the way to create the best public services for the money spent:

Our preference is that power over the public services that people use as individuals should go to those individuals wherever possible. No one knows an individual's preferences better than they do, and while some people may need extra help to choose the services they want, at the centre of our vision is the belief that people should be trusted to choose the best services for themselves rather than being forced to accept choices determined by others. (HM Government, 2011, p 14)

The White Paper distinguishes between areas where there is some public benefit in the government setting limits on how public money is used by individuals and areas where individuals are best placed to choose how best to meet their needs. For the former, vouchers and per capita funding such as the Pupil Premium in education are the most appropriate mechanisms. For the latter, the White Paper identifies a huge opportunity to shift power to individuals through individual budgets, delivered as cash payments where possible. The initiatives across government outside the Department of Health that are seeking to accelerate the transfer of power to individuals through individual budgets are described here.

Right to Control Trailblazers, Department for Work and Pensions

As well as receiving support from adult social care, many disabled people access a range of other services that are the responsibility of other government departments, such as support for employment through the Department for Work and Pension's Access to Work scheme. The Right to Control Trailblazers are seeking to maximise choice and control for individuals with disabilities by providing them with a single integrated individual budget across six funding streams from three different Whitehall departments: Access to Work, Work Choice, Disabled Facilities Grant, Independent Living Fund, Adult Social Care and Supporting People. The centrepiece of this attempt at integration is a legal right for individuals to request that their services and supports be delivered in an integrated way and through an individual budget if they choose – the individual right to control.

There are seven Right to Control Trailblazer local authorities or local authority partnerships that started implementation in 2010 and were intended to finish by the end of 2012. Given limited progress by the end of 2011, the Trailblazers were extended until December 2013 in order to give areas more time for implementation. An early process evaluation found that most disabled individuals were unaware of their 'right to control', and staff also lacked awareness and understanding of the approach. However, staff were more positive that the Right to Control was encouraging partnership working across services, even if there was some way to go to make the approach mainstream. Pulling together different funding streams into a single budget is a major challenge, particularly in an environment of significant cuts to public spending. The Trailblazers face an ongoing tension between making the individual right meaningful, while ensuring sustainability and fair access for all (Tu et al, 2012).

Special educational needs and disability pathfinders, Department for Education

Running alongside the PHB pilot which focused on adults with long-term health needs has been a parallel initiative for children which was launched in the 2011 Green Paper, *Support and aspiration: A new approach to special educational needs and disability* (DfE, 2011). From April 2014, parents of children with special educational needs and disabilities (SEND) will have the right for their child to have a single assessment across education, health and social services, a single plan from zero to 25 years of age and to control parts of that plan through an individual budget.

This approach is being tested over an 18-month period in 20 pathfinder sites consisting of 31 local authorities and their health partners in order to inform wider national roll-out. The SEND pathfinders build on an earlier pilot of budget-holding lead professionals for disabled children (HM Treasury and DfES, 2005) and several high profile examples of the use of individual budgets for young people in transition to adult services (see Epilogue). An interim evaluation at the half-way point concluded that the pathfinders had not made the speed of progress anticipated, with individual budgets being one of the least developed aspects (Craston et al, 2012). As this and the evaluation of the Right to Control initiative highlight, implementation of individual budget programmes is always challenging. They require new infrastructure, new ways of working and a complete culture change, all of which take time to develop and implement.

Rough sleepers, Department for Communities and Local Government

One of the smaller individual budget initiatives was the pilot undertaken by the homelessness charity, Broadway, for long-term rough sleepers as part of the City of London Corporation and Department for Communities and Local Government's strategy to end rough sleeping. Each of the 21 rough sleepers had a budget of up to £3,000 and was allocated a broker with whom to develop a plan to move off the streets.

Of the 21 participants, 16 moved into accommodation and a further three were awaiting accommodation offers at the end of the evaluation. This is an impressive record of success given that some of the participants had been on the streets for up to 45 years. Participants spent less than they were allocated, £794 on average. As with all other individual budget programmes, the personalised plan was found to be as significant in the pilot's success as the budget itself. As the evaluation concludes, 'the personalised approach has brought people elements of choice and control not provided by standard offers of support, alongside intensive support from one trusted worker' (Hough and Rice, 2010, p 1). The pilot ended in 2011, but individual budgets have been incorporated into Broadway's standard way of working with rough sleepers in the City of London.

Personalisation and public service integration

One of the ongoing challenges for public services is how to integrate to meet the needs of those who rely on more than one service. For example, one in eight budget holders and a majority of carers in the PHB evaluation also received social care funding (Forder et al, 2012). All too often, users of multiple services find themselves retelling their story at each assessment and review. They have to disentangle their lives to fit the bureaucratic boundaries of services, and either find that support from different services duplicates or they fall through the gaps between services. At the same time, they present a significant cost to government that is only increased by a disjointed service response.

Clearly, there is a risk that, as personalisation expands across public services, individuals end up with multiple budgets to manage that are not integrated to provide whole person support. However, the expansion of personalisation also provides an important opportunity to accelerate integration across public services, with different funding streams contributing to a single individual budget. System-level integration – bringing organisations together, pooling budgets and developing joint posts – has been the traditional route to integration, but its success has been limited and progress tends to unravel in tough financial times. When budgets are tight, organisations see greater interest in defending their own turf than in collaborating. Take the NHS and social care, as an example. Despite 40 years of efforts to coordinate resources across the two systems, less than 5 per cent of the combined NHS and social care budgets are spent through joint funding arrangements (Humphries and Curry, 2011). Furthermore, integration at the organisational level does not guarantee a joined-up experience of services for the individual. Starting from the point of view of the individual is more likely to lead to an integrated experience, in large part because individuals have the strongest incentives to ensure that their support is well coordinated (Glendinning et al, 2000b; Miller et al, 2011).

Of course, integration across funding streams at the individual level is not straightforward, as the challenges facing the Right to Control Trailblazers and SEND pathfinders demonstrate. A previous attempt in 2005 at implementing integrated individual budgets for people with disabilities – the individual budget pilot – also hit up against the challenges of coordinating funding streams that have different eligibility criteria, narrowly defined purposes and where accountability for spending remains with the original government department (Glendinning et al, 2008).

However, the challenges appear more surmountable if a 'dual carriageway' approach can be adopted that leaves organisational structures in place. This involves bringing together the referral, assessment, budget setting, planning and monitoring of different budgets without the complexities of structural integration between organisations and government departments. The individual experiences the benefits of a single system, although behind the scenes, the systems remain separate (NHS Confederation, 2012).

Over the last decade, personalisation has become an important strand of public service reform and, as this chapter has highlighted, there is now considerable activity across government to introduce individual budgets, and between government departments to develop integrated individual budgets. Seen in this context, the decision to introduce PHBs into the NHS is not an isolated reform but part of a broader strand of thinking reshaping the relationship between the state, public service professionals and citizens to recognise the importance of individual choice and control in securing the best possible outcomes from investment in public services. The remaining chapters in this section turn to PHBs specifically. The next chapter provides an introduction to

PHBs and the five ways in which they contribute to the development of a truly patient-centred NHS.

TWO

What is a personal health budget? The basics explained

A PHB is a new way of meeting health needs that is highly responsive to individuals but respects the principles of the NHS that access to care is based on need and is free at the point of use. At its simplest, a PHB is an amount of NHS funding which is allocated to an individual to meet a health need that satisfies existing NHS criteria for support instead of receiving centrally commissioned services. The PHB allows individuals or their carers on their behalf to choose how best to meet their health needs. For example, Colin's family found that renting a flat and buying a Sky Plus box was a far more effective approach to managing their father Malcolm's behaviour, as his dementia progressed, than the NHS day service to which he had originally been referred. Since he was unhappy at the day service, his behaviour became worse. Soon, four staff were needed to manage him and his medication had to be increased. He is now on a third of the medication he was on then and on his lowest level since coming out of hospital four years ago. Malcolm's PHB has also enabled him to keep living at home four years after his family was told that he would never live at home again.

The five essential features of a personal health budget
According to the Department of Health, the following are the five essential features of a PHB. The person with the PHB (or their representative) will:

- be able to choose the health and wellbeing outcomes they want to achieve, in agreement with a healthcare professional;
- know how much money they have for their healthcare and support;
- be enabled to create their own care plan, with support if they want it;
- be able to choose how their budget is held and managed, including the right to ask for a direct payment;
- be able to spend the money in ways and at times that makes sense to them, as agreed in their plan.

Source: DH (2012e)

PHBs are not appropriate for all aspects of healthcare. In an emergency, few people want to make choices about their treatment. They want to hand over those decisions to a well-trained expert whose skills can help them survive. However, the majority of healthcare spending in the UK and in other developed economies is now related to the ongoing management of long-term conditions for people living at home (Alakeson and Rosen, 2011). This is where PHBs come into their own. Long-term conditions such as depression, chronic obstructive pulmonary disorder (COPD) and multiple sclerosis (MS) shape people's day-to-day experiences, and ongoing management of these conditions has to be compatible with people's lives. As such, the response from the NHS needs to be as personal as possible to be effective, and this requires people being in control of how best to meet their needs. Achieving the same clinical outcomes as a passive recipient of care would contribute less to that individual's wellbeing and quality of life (Sen, 2001, 2010). This is well demonstrated by the results of the national PHB evaluation that found significant improvements in care-related quality of life from the exercise of individual choice and control (Forder et al, 2012). The evaluation results are discussed in more detail in Chapter 5.

Personal health budgets and a patient-led NHS

The current Coalition government has made 'no decision about me, without me' the defining concept of its proposals for NHS reform, and the subsequent 2012 Health and Social Care Act. PHBs are central to the government's intention to create a patient-led NHS. As Andrew Lansley wrote in his Secretary of State's 2012 annual report:

> If managed well, people with long-term conditions may not need to be treated within secondary care but, too often, care is uncoordinated and does not fit in with the individual's life, leading to a crisis point and a hospital admission. Instead, personalisation, empowerment and shared decision-making, for example through expanding patient choice, personalised care planning and personal health budgets, will help people to have far greater input into decisions about their care, and more control over the care they receive including where and when they receive it. This also offers greater potential for self-management and self-care, where the person is empowered to manage their condition. (Lansley, 2012, p 14)

PHBs support the creation of a patient-led NHS by radically changing how the NHS operates to align more closely with the ways in which users of the NHS view their health, how health fits with the rest of their life and their motivations for improving their health. PHBs do this in five specific ways. They:

- allow individuals to choose how their needs are met and break out of the limitations of centrally commissioned services;
- recognise individuals as experts in their own condition and bring the service user experience into the care planning process;
- promote a social model of health that recognises that health cannot be separated from other aspects of people's lives and improving health needs to go beyond healthcare;
- focus on including people within society, not just purchasing alternative services;
- allow a real transfer of power to take place within the NHS through the individual control of resources, and do not pay lip service to partnership.

The rest of this chapter discusses each of these five dimensions of PHBs and the ways in which they transform the delivery of care in the NHS. While other approaches to changing practice in the NHS such as shared decision making share common ground with PHBs, as discussed in Chapter 4, these five features together make PHBs a unique and powerful tool for change.

Extending patient choice

The 2009 NHS Constitution enshrines the right for individuals to make choices about their NHS care and to receive information to support these choices. At present, this right only extends as far as choosing which organisation provides care when individuals are referred for their first outpatient appointment with a consultant-led service. Surveys indicate that people value choice far more highly than clinicians, with clinicians often believing that patients already have adequate choice (NMHDU, 2011a). In one survey, 75 per cent of respondents said choice was either 'very important' or 'important' to them. Older respondents, those with no qualifications, and those from a mixed and non-white background were more likely to value choice, challenging the assumption that choice is the preserve of the better off and better educated (Dixon et al, 2010). As well as choice of provider, there is evidence that individuals would like to change elements of their care package but are not optimistic about being able to do so (NMHDU, 2011b).

For the first time in the NHS, PHBs give people choices about how their health needs are met as well as where their care is delivered, by whom and at what time. They make people commissioners in their own right and allow them to be creative and to tailor their care to their very personal circumstances. For some, simply changing provider or having greater control over when care is delivered can make a significant difference to their life. For others, the flexibility to meet their needs in ways that break out of the confines of traditionally commissioned services is more valuable. For example, Martin has motor neurone disease and uses part of his PHB to make a weekly trip to the barbers to have his hair washed and his beard trimmed, something that the traditional NHS would never provide. Presenting himself well despite his condition is important to Martin's self-esteem and improves his wellbeing. By going to the barbers, that is one less task for his wife and children, helping to sustain them in their caring role, and the trip to the barbers stops him becoming isolated at home and depressed (DH, 2011b). Put together, it all helps to maintain his current level of independence, preventing him from deteriorating further and needing more expensive NHS services.

Decisions about how best to use the resources in a PHB are made through a care planning process that is led by individuals in collaboration with their clinicians, family and with independent support if they choose. Through this process, individuals identify what works well and not so well about their current care and support, the goals they have for their health and wellbeing and how those goals can be met.

The Department of Health has identified only a small number of things that a PHB cannot be used to buy. A range of NHS services are excluded: GP services, NHS charges, public health services such as immunisations, prescription medications, operations, emergency services and any other unplanned care. In addition, a PHB cannot be used for alcohol, cigarettes, gambling, debt repayments and anything illegal because these represent an inappropriate use of public money (DH, 2013). Beyond this, there is no set menu, and commissioners should resist imposing one. The national evaluation found that restrictive approaches to implementing PHBs led to poorer outcomes for budget holders than flexible approaches that promoted creativity (Forder et al, 2012). The Sky Plus Box mentioned earlier would never have appeared on a list of service options for dementia that had been pre-determined by commissioners. Yet it has been highly effective for Malcolm and his family. Its effectiveness stems from the fact that it is a personalised solution. Table 2.1 shows the diversity of purchases that individuals made with their PHBs in the first nine months of the national pilot programme.

Recognising the expertise of individuals

While clinical professionals are experts in the scientific evidence related to particular conditions and have significant knowledge about how individuals respond to different treatments, they cannot know the priorities that each person has for his or her care. Only individuals and their families have access to this knowledge and can know the trade-offs they would make between different possible outcomes, for example, being pain-free compared to being too drowsy from painkillers to work. Traditional models of clinical training and practice

Table 2.1: Use of personal health budgets at nine months

Types of use	Examples
Care	Employing carers or personal assistants, respite care
Physical healthcare treatments	Physiotherapy, neuro-physiotherapy, speech therapy, occupational therapy
Healthcare or personal care equipment	Nebuliser, sanitary equipment, aprons and rubber gloves
Psychological therapies and counselling	Neuro-linguistic sessions, counselling
Alternative or complementary therapies	Acupuncture, Reiki, massage, reflexology, yoga, Chinese medicine, bio-neuro therapy
Cosmetic/beauty treatments	Manicure, hair removal, hairdresser
Physical exercise	Gym membership, exercise classes, home exercise equipment, personal training
Improved dietary management	Frozen meals delivered, dietetics sessions
Computers/technology	Laptop, mobile phone, satellite navigation device, emergency 999 telecare system
Aids and adaptations	Wheelchair, adjustable armchair, adjustable table
Facilitating social activities and hobbies	Season ticket, craft materials, musical instrument, driving lessons, childcare, clothes, activity day with friends, theatre trip
Domestic help	Gardener, cleaner
Domestic appliances	Fridge, freezer, blender
Travel/transport	Travel to/from gym, travel for husband to make hospital visits, mobility scooter
Administration fees	Providers of employment administrative support (taxation, National Insurance), staff training

Source: Davidson et al (2012, p 13)

are predicated on professional expertise alone and the expectation that clinicians will make recommendations and identify solutions for their patients. However, without taking individual preferences into consideration, treatment is unlikely to be successful. The World Health Organization estimates that between 30 and 50 per cent of patients, depending on the condition, do not take their prescribed medicines as recommended (WHO, 2003). Furthermore, outcomes are likely to be more positive if individuals feel actively engaged as partners in their own care (Epstein et al, 2010).

By giving control to individuals, PHBs recognise that the successful management of long-term conditions and disabilities requires bringing together the learned expertise of professionals with the lived experiences of individuals and families. This is the central principle of shared decision making in healthcare (Coulter and Collins, 2011). As Deegan and Drake (2006) explain, it is in bringing together these two types of expertise and experimenting that effective solutions can be found.

> Shared decision making diverges radically from compliance because it assumes two experts – the client and the practitioner – must share respective information and determine collaboratively optimum treatment…. It helps to bridge the empirical evidence base, which is established on population averages, with the unique concerns, values and life context of the individual client. From the vantage point of the individual healthcare client, the efficacy of a particular medication is not certain … the question of how the medication will affect the individual becomes an open experiment for two co-experimenters – the client and the practitioner. (Deegan and Drake, 2006, p 1636)

The concept of shared decision making was developed in the context of clinical decision making. For example, a woman who has been diagnosed with breast cancer may have to make a range of treatment decisions such as whether to have a lumpectomy or a mastectomy and whether to have chemotherapy or only radiotherapy. Shared decision making aims to equip her and her clinician to have a more equal and more informed conversation about these choices. It is in this clinical context that her priorities, preferences and social situation matter. PHBs build on the philosophy of shared decision making but broaden the context beyond clinical care to focus on quality of life, as discussed next.

Adopting a social model of health

The NHS has its roots in a medical model of health which views health as the absence of disease and disease as the result of dysfunction in the body. While models of long-term conditions management have started to recognise the importance of wider social factors (Wagner, 1998), the NHS is still largely focused on managing and meeting narrowly defined healthcare needs related to specific diagnoses. It measures its success on the basis of symptom management, improvements in clinical functions such as blood glucose levels, reductions in hospital admissions and survival rates. These are important outcomes and it is right that the NHS should strive to match the best in the world, but these measures tell us little about an individual's quality of life and their ability to pursue the other roles in life that matter most to them, such as being a parent or a successful business person. We do not hold the NHS to account for how many people with long-term health conditions continue to work, or even expect that to be a consideration for a health service, although it is often the main priority for the people receiving care.

According to Crisp (2010), the consumption of healthcare in affluent countries has become an end in itself rather than the means to a better life. In low-income countries where resources are scarce, healthcare remains focused on helping people to regain their capacity to earn a living. PHBs attempt to reconnect healthcare to the whole person and their wider social context, not just to treat a diagnosis. They aim to address health needs in order to ensure that people can enjoy a good quality of life and be productive members of society.

Too often, NHS care works inadvertently against other important parts of people's lives, as Tom discovered when he sustained a spinal cord injury from a snowboarding accident and was assessed as needing 24-hour care from a specialist agency. The care got in the way of his job that requires government security clearance for him and his carers. The carers moved on more quickly than their clearance could be processed which restricted the projects Tom could work on, affecting his overall quality of life. Despite having the specialist skills required by the healthcare regulator, the agency was not focused on delivering care that enabled Tom to carry on with the rest of his life. He tried to negotiate with the agency but was not making much progress when the idea of a PHB came up. He decided to stick with the same agency because they provide highly specialised care for people with spinal injuries, but his PHB allowed him to become the direct purchaser of his care, giving him more influence over the agency. This has helped to improve the quality and continuity of his care.

Focusing on social inclusion

Although PHBs are part of the suite of NHS reforms that rely on the market to diversify provision and change provider behaviour, their ultimate focus is not on fostering consumerism but on rebuilding people's rights to full inclusion in society. All too often, the lives of individuals with significant health needs become dominated by specialist services. They become isolated from their communities, retreat from universal services and even their social interaction is reduced to group-based activities run by NHS services. Their needs are met, but only in the narrowest of senses. They are stuck in 'service land' rather than being active participants in their communities.

PHBs are not just a means of replacing NHS services with alternatives purchased from elsewhere. The care planning process considers how all resources within the community can be marshalled to meet individual outcomes. They aim to reconnect people who have become isolated within specialist services with their communities, and in doing so, help maintain health and wellbeing. Alex's experience provides a good illustration of how a PHB can act as a bridge to new relationships and a renewed purpose. Alex suffered a stroke that left him mildly physically and cognitively disabled and very depressed. Despite receiving services from his community mental health team for his depression, he only started to make progress towards recovery when he began attending a peer support group for stroke survivors that helped reduce his isolation. When he then got a PHB, his life really started to change. He used his PHB to buy a satellite navigation device to help him drive to medical appointments without getting lost. The stroke had affected his short-term memory, making it difficult for him to remember directions, but driving helped him concentrate. With the navigation device, he was able to get himself around and, more importantly, offer lifts to other people in his peer support group, making him feel useful again and allowing him to feel that he was giving something back. As a result of finding a new community and building new relationships, Alex's mental health has improved and he now rarely sees his community mental health team. In an interview, he described his experience of having a PHB as follows:

> 'Twelve months ago I would have been quite happy to die. Now I help other people. I'm paying my bit back. By giving me financial help [through a PHB], the NHS has done its bit, now I am trying to give back by volunteering at the Stroke Association and for peer support groups. The

PHB was very instrumental in changing my life. The things
I bought may seem frivolous but they really work.'

As in Alex's case, PHBs can be the catalyst to building reciprocal
networks of support for people and, in doing so, can enhance their
'real wealth' – the set of things in addition to money that contribute
to a good life such as access to community, human relationships and
opportunities to use one's talents (Murray and Duffy, 2011). PHBs
can be pooled across individuals to help support group activities and
reduce isolation. There are several good examples of individuals pooling
personal budgets in social care that offer a model for PHBs as they
develop. The members of Re-energise, an Oxford-based sports and
social group run by users of mental health services, decided to pool
their personal budgets to sustain the group after its start-up funding
came to an end (NMHDU, 2010). Ealing Centre for Independent
Living supported a group of 25 people with learning difficulties to pool
their personal budgets to pay for a theatre course they had previously
attended when the college decided to withdraw it (NCIL, 2008).

Part of the contribution of PHBs to social inclusion stems from a
more holistic planning process which recognises that, however much
support people may need, they also have a contribution to make. The
medical model generally recognises people's diagnoses and deficits.
Assessments are based on what an individual cannot do and rarely
capture the assets they bring to their own health improvement and the
roles they could meaningfully fulfil. By putting individuals in control,
PHBs start from a different place. As the Equality and Human Rights
Commissioner, Baroness Jane Campbell, said of her own disability in
an interview with the *Daily Telegraph* in 2012, 'it is very difficult to
accept charity. I don't want to be somebody's good cause. It is much
easier when people recognise that you have something to give them
in return' (quoted in Moreton, 2012).

Tipping the balance of power

The four dimensions of PHBs that have already been discussed in this
chapter are dependent on the fifth dimension that is unique to PHBs:
PHBs transfer control of NHS resources to individuals and families.
In doing so, they genuinely shift the balance of power in the NHS
to make a reality of partnership, and reorient services away from the
medical model.

There is good evidence that if a PHB was nothing more than money,
it would not help meet people's needs in better ways (Brewis et al, 2012).

The care planning process that supports people to identify how they want to spend their money is critical and is discussed in more detail in Section 2 of this book. At the same time, giving individuals control by allocating NHS resources to them makes it harder for professionals and service providers to pay lip service to partnership, while seeking to retain control. With resources in their hands, it is easier for individuals and families to feel on an equal footing with professionals than if the partnership depended on the good will of professionals alone.

Furthermore, by creating transparency around how much is available to individuals, the PHB process enables them to plan effectively. In the traditional NHS, patients have no idea how much money is spent on their care, and few clinicians know how much services cost. PHB holders have been shocked to discover that thousands had previously been spent on care that they did not consider good value for money. Knowing how much there is to spend allows individuals to maximise their creativity and encourages them to pursue value for money (Forder et al, 2012, p 163). They have to prioritise and make choices in order to meet their needs within their allocated budget. For example, if a person had two goals, to re-establish a relationship with family overseas and to return to work, it might make more sense for them to use their PHB for a computer microphone and webcam so that they could call family for free over the internet, leaving them money to pay for retraining rather than going to visit family in person. Without knowing how much there is to spend, it is impossible to prioritise in this way.

PHBs are a new way of delivering NHS services, but they are also a tool to radically transform the NHS away from a professionally dominated, medical model of healthcare to one that values the expertise of individuals and that seeks to support them to meet their health needs in ways that respect the other things that matter in their lives. The next chapter explores where PHBs have come from, and traces the development of personalisation from social care into the NHS.

THREE

The development of personalisation: from direct payments to personal health budgets

The decision to pilot PHBs in the NHS in England in 2009 can be traced back through a series of actors and events to the 1980s when disabled people, inspired by their peers in the US, started organising to move out of institutional care. However, there is not a straight line linking the campaigns of disabled people for independent living to PHBs. Rather, a set of related initiatives and interactions between disabled people, their allies, researchers and policymakers accounts for developments over the last 30 years. This chapter charts these developments to put PHBs in historical context.

Independent living and direct payments

Until the 1980s it was common for disabled people to be segregated from the rest of society in large institutional settings. At worst, these were hostile, abusive environments, more akin to prisons than a home. At best, they offered a uniform approach to care that left little room to cater to individual needs or preferences (Arnold, 2010). While recent abuse scandals have highlighted the importance of sustained pressure for quality improvement in residential care (DH, 2012a), services for disabled people are now oriented around supporting people to live as part of the wider community. The campaign for 'independent living' and the end of institutional care was pioneered by disabled people in the US whose influence spread to campaigners in the UK and in the rest of Europe. It took nearly 30 years, but the last long-stay institution for people with learning disabilities in the UK closed in 2009 (Mencap, 2009).

Within the disability movement, 'independent living' is defined as 'all disabled people having the same choice, control and freedom as any other citizen – at home, at work, and as members of the community' (DRC, 2002). A parallel movement made similar demands on behalf of people with mental health problems who were also consigned to appalling long-stay institutions. Like the 'independent living' movement, the 'recovery' movement was born out of the lived experience of people who had faced the challenge of living with and growing beyond a diagnosis of mental health problems (O'Hagan, 1993; Deegan, 1997). Recovery focuses on supporting and enabling people to lead flourishing and fulfilling lives as part of their communities, regardless of their mental health problems.

The closure of long-stay institutions was, however, not the end of the independent living campaign or recovery movement. Having left institutions, many disabled found themselves living in the community but trapped within segregated, specialist services and denied the opportunity to play a full part in family and community life, as discussed in the last chapter. This led to further calls for independence and control that were expressed most clearly in the direct payments campaign launched by the British Council of Disabled People in 1989.

In the 1980s, a small number of disabled people in Hampshire were able to hire their own personal assistants through a cash payment instead of receiving services commissioned by the local authority. However, the 1948 Social Security Act was ambiguous as to whether or not it was legal for local authorities to offer these direct payments. This ambiguity can be traced back to the eradication of the 1834 Poor Law and the creation of the welfare state that separated the idea of social care from social security. Following the eradication of the Poor Law, social care and social work professionals were no longer concerned with poverty and cash assistance. Income support became the realm of social security. In this context, the introduction of direct payments was seen as a step backwards and a blurring of the boundary between social care services and income support (Glasby and Littlechild, 2002). In 1992, Virginia Bottomley, the Minister for Health at the time, ruled that 'direct payments' were illegal.

The direct payments campaign set out to change the law to make direct payments available to all disabled people. It was spurred on by the growth of centres for independent living, an idea that started in California and had at its heart the concept of personal assistants working directly for disabled people (Zarb and Nadash, 1994). The campaign was also boosted by the popularity of the Independent Living Fund that was established in 1986 to provide cash assistance to disabled people to purchase personal assistance services. By 1993, the Fund was serving 22,000 people at a cost of £82 million compared to its original budget of £5 million (Morris, 1993). After a five-year effort supported by a Private Members Bill and independent research, direct payments were made legal in 1997 and in 2003, it became mandatory for local authorities to offer them to all those who were eligible and who requested one (Evans, 2003).

Personalisation as policy

The development of personalisation as a strand of policy thinking in social care drew on the independent living movement and its campaign for direct payments, but was also shaped by think tanks, policymakers, politicians and the professional allies of disabled people, as well as developments internationally. The term itself was first coined by the commentator Charles Leadbeater in 2004 to describe a range of developments aimed at empowering users of public services to become equal 'co-producers' of decisions with professionals and service providers (Leadbeater, 2004). Policymakers gravitated towards personalisation and individual control of services because of the possibility of savings. Research commissioned from the Policy Studies Institute for the direct payments campaign had demonstrated 30 to 40 per cent savings over commissioned services (Zarb and Nadash, 1994), and Germany's cash for care scheme awarded individuals who chose the cash payment option only 50 per cent of the value of in-kind services without leaving them unable to meet their needs (Alakeson, 2010). The 2005 individual budgets pilot demonstrated improvements in cost-effectiveness rather than absolute savings, but allayed fears about cost growth (Glendinning et al, 2008).

Perhaps the strongest influence on the evolution of personalisation in social care came from the work of In Control, a social enterprise that developed the concept of a personal budget. Despite the long fight to make direct payments a reality, they were criticised because the amount available through a direct payment was based on the service package an individual would otherwise have received. This left most of the anomalies of the existing system in place, with people having similar levels of need receiving vastly different amounts of money depending on their disability. In Control reversed the system, creating an upfront allocation of resources based on need that the individual could choose how best to use through a support planning process. Direct payments became one route through which individuals could choose to manage their personal budget, with different third party management options also possible. By providing third party management options, personal budgets opened up choice and control to many more people who did not want the responsibility of a direct payment.

Putting People First and the mainstreaming of personal budgets

In December 2007, *Putting People First* brought personalisation into the policy mainstream for adult social care in a ministerial concordat agreed between central and local government, the sector's professional leadership, providers and the regulator (HM Government, 2007). The centrepiece of the policy was the proposal to give everyone eligible for publicly funded adult social care access to a personal budget which they could use to meet their agreed social care outcomes. *Putting People First* recognised that personal budgets needed to be supported by a wider set of changes to make a reality of personalisation in adult social care. For example, if personal budgets were not to become an add-on, adult social care would have to start recognising people with support needs as assets who could make a positive contribution to their local communities and would have to work to change universal and other commercial services to allow people to become less reliant on specialist, targeted services.

The implementation of personal budgets was initially driven by a national target for 30 per cent of all service users with ongoing care and support needs in each local authority to have a personal budget by April 2011. In its 2010 adult social care strategy, the government raised the stakes, setting an ambitious target of having all council-funded service users and carers on personal budgets by April 2013, with as many as possible using direct payments (DH, 2010b). This target was superseded in 2012 by the Draft Care and Support Bill which creates an entitlement to a personal budget for all social care users and carers who meet eligibility criteria (Secretary of State for Health, 2012).

Self-directed support is the mechanism and framework through which personal budgets are delivered (Glasby and Littlechild, 2009). Self-directed support involves finding out what is important to people with social care needs and their families and friends, and helping them to plan how to use the available money to achieve these aims. It is about focusing on outcomes and ensuring that people have choice and control over their support arrangements. Many of the steps in the personal health budget process described in Section 2 draw on self-directed support.

Self-directed support in social care

Implementing self-directed support in social care involves the following seven steps:

Step 1: Allocating the money. The first step is to identify the resources to be made available to the individual to achieve his or her outcomes. At this stage, this is an indicative allocation that will be finalised in Step 3 following the development of a support plan.

Step 2: Developing a support plan. The second step is for individuals to put together a plan for how they will use the money allocated to get the life they want. The plan can include broader needs and desired outcomes beyond those that made the person eligible for support. Support plans should not be constrained by the menu of services currently offered. The plan can be completed by individuals themselves or with support, but their voice must be central.

Step 3: Getting the support plan agreed. The plan has to be approved by a local authority social worker to confirm that it is appropriate to meet the objectives identified by the individual, that it is safe and within budget.

Step 4: Organising the money. Once the plan is approved, the personal budget allocation is finalised and individuals can decide whether to manage the money as a direct payment or to have it managed for them. A combination of the two is also possible.

Step 5: Putting the support in place. Individuals can organise the support approved in their plans in ways that suit them and the rest of their lives. This means that providers have to be more flexible in responding to individual needs. Individuals can look beyond specialist services for support, drawing on goods, universal services and people they know to support them.

Step 6: Living life. With the right support in place, individuals can live the best life possible and pursue the goals they have set out in their plans.

Step 7: Reviewing how things worked. The local authority should have a process for checking at least annually whether the outcomes agreed in the support plan have been achieved. Individuals also have to demonstrate that the money has been used as planned.

Sources: Adapted from In Control's Seven Steps (www.in-control.org.uk/support/support-for-individuals,-family-members-carers/seven-steps-to-being-in-control.aspx) and ADASS and South West Regional Improvement and Efficiency Partnership (2010).

By 2012, 53 per cent of eligible users of adult social care services in England – around 432,000 people – had a personal budget, an increase of 38 per cent on the previous year. Progress has been much slower in Scotland and Wales, with fewer than 5,000 people on a direct payment in 2011 in Scotland and fewer than 3,000 people in Wales. Implementation has been highly variable across local authorities within England and between different disability groups. As of 2012, 7 per cent of councils were still falling short of the 2011 target, with fewer than a quarter of eligible individuals on a personal budget, although this fell from 26 per cent in 2011 (ADASS, 2012). Take-up has always been highest among younger people with physical and learning disabilities. Take-up in England in 2010-11 was 41 per cent among working-age adults with a learning disability and 35 per cent of physically disabled adults of working age, compared to 29 per cent of older people. People with mental health problems continue to lag behind, with only 9 per cent using a personal budget (Samuel, 2012).

Evaluations of self-directed models internationally consistently reveal a positive picture despite significant differences in programme design (Alakeson, 2010). The strongest findings relate to improvements in satisfaction with services and improvements in quality of life (discussed in greater detail in Chapter 4). However, the 2011 National Personal Budget Survey of 2,000 personal budget users and carers in England did reveal how differences in implementation across local authorities affect individual outcomes, much as the national PHB evaluation found (Forder et al, 2012). Outcomes were better where individuals were informed about the value of their personal budget, fully involved in the support planning process alongside family members, were relatively free of constraints and bureaucracy, and where their support was managed through a direct payment rather than a council-managed budget (Hatton and Waters, 2011). These issues will be discussed later in this chapter when we explore how lessons from social care can inform the implementation of PHBs.

From personal budgets in social care to personal health budgets

It has long been recognised that the point at which we divide the NHS from social care is little more than a bureaucratic boundary between service systems and has no intrinsic logic. The Health Select Committee concluded that:

… the question of what is health and what is social care is one to which we can find no satisfactory answer, and which our witnesses were similarly unable to explain in meaningful terms…. We strongly recommend that the Government remove once and for all the wholly artificial distinction between a universal and free health care service operating alongside a means-tested and charged for system of social care. (House of Commons Health Committee, 2005)

Furthermore, evidence emerged early on in the implementation of direct payments that individuals were using their social care funds to pay for goods and services that would traditionally have been defined as NHS care such as injections, dressings and nursing care. They had little regard for the boundary between services and simply sought to coordinate the care they needed in the best way possible (Glendinning et al, 2000a).

The development of personal budgets and their positive impact on people's lives, therefore, raised the question as to whether the approach should be extended into those areas of the NHS that address long-term health needs (Glasby and Hasler, 2004; Glasby, 2008). Of all the possible areas, NHS continuing healthcare (CHC) was the one where the need for a more personalised approach was most pressing. Approximately 56,000 people with long-term, complex health needs receive CHC, and a significant proportion transition into CHC from social care. Prior to the extension of PHBs to anyone eligible for CHC, people who qualified for NHS care were forced to give up the control they had enjoyed through a social care direct payment. This left individuals and families distressed, reduced the quality of care they received and limited their quality of life.

The extension of personalisation into the NHS was initially fiercely resisted for several reasons. First, healthcare was viewed as more complex and specialist than social care and an area where clinical professionals rather than individuals were experts. Second, as with other types of choice in healthcare, there were concerns that PHBs would exacerbate health inequalities by working in favour of the better off and better educated, and third, there were fears that costs would increase as PHBs would draw people into the NHS who would not want traditional services (Dixon and Ashton, 2008). Perhaps the greatest concern was that PHBs would violate the basic principles of the NHS and leave open the possibility of top-ups, with individuals adding their own money to an NHS PHB (Lewis, 2011). There was also a practical stumbling block: until the introduction of the PHB pilot and its accompanying legislation, it was illegal for the NHS to pay money to citizens.

Despite these barriers, PHBs had some influential supporters such as former Secretary of State for Health, Alan Milburn (2007), Downing Street adviser Professor Julian Le Grand (2007) and Lord Darzi, the Minister of Health in charge of the 2008 NHS Next Stage Review. His final report, *High quality care for all*, proposed piloting PHBs (DH, 2008). Despite resistance from medical organisations and trade unions, a three-year pilot was implemented in 2009. As discussed in the Introduction to this book, the government has since committed to the expansion of PHBs, starting with individuals eligible for CHC from April 2014. Figure 3.1 shows how the concepts we have discussed in this chapter are nested, one inside the other, starting with independent living and ending with PHBs.

Figure 3.1: The conceptual history of personal health budgets (PHBs)

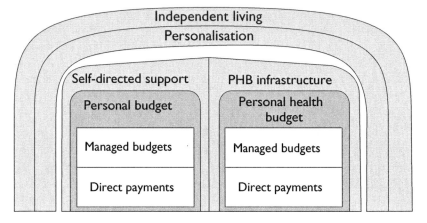

Lessons from social care

In the last couple of years, concerns about the ways in which personalisation has progressed in social care have led some of its original advocates to back away from it (Duffy, 2011a; SCIE and nef, 2011). Their view is that the individual empowerment that was integral to the approach has been lost through underfunding and poor implementation. Five years on from *Putting People First*, now is a good time to look to social care for lessons to inform the expansion of PHBs. Many of the challenges that local authority commissioners continue to grapple with are the same ones that NHS commissioners will confront as PHBs roll out. The remainder of this chapter discusses the following five lessons from the implementation of personal budgets in adult social care:

• Decommissioning services to enable real choice and control is essential.
• The availability of support services is critical to making personalisation inclusive.
• Bureaucracy should be limited to protect individual empowerment.
• Culture change takes time and needs real investment.
• Implementation will vary dramatically without a national approach.

Decommissioning services

Although the numbers with a personal budget continue to rise, much of this increase is in council-managed budgets rather than direct payments. The percentage opting for a direct payment has stagnated at 26 per cent of personal budgets since 2010, despite a stated policy preference for direct payments (ADASS, 2012). This is cause for concern because evaluations have clearly demonstrated that direct payments lead to far greater choice and control than council-managed budgets (Routledge and Lewis, 2011). This is largely because direct payments provide individuals with greater flexibility and allow them to use their personal budget as they choose, for example, to hire their own personal assistants. Council-managed budgets have been implemented in such a way as to restrict individuals to the services that have already been commissioned by the local authority or, at best where the council has a framework agreement in place, to a list of pre-selected providers. The result is that many people who have a council-managed budget have seen no real change in the services they receive and experience little additional choice and control. The only difference is that they know how much money is being spent on their services.

Of course, council-managed budgets are not, by their very nature, restrictive. They can be used flexibly. But they have been implemented in a restrictive way in many local authorities because much of the money available to fund community-based services remains tied up in block-purchased contracts. Without undoing these contracts and decommissioning existing services, there is not enough unallocated money available to offer all personal budget holders free choice of how they use their budget. For example, if all of the council's resources for adult social care are tied up in contracts with four large domiciliary care agencies, individuals who get a personal budget can choose to switch from one agency to another, but there is not enough money outside of these existing contracts to allow budget holders to hire their own personal assistants, which they might prefer.

This issue of decommissioning services is common to the NHS and social care. As PHBs are rolled out, their sustainability and ability to deliver real change for individuals, particularly those who do not want the responsibility of managing a direct payment, will depend on the extent to which existing services can be decommissioned to unlock funding for PHBs. Decommissioning is discussed in greater detail in Section 3. Failure to decommission services as PHBs expand will result in the NHS replicating the split system currently operating in social care where, for large numbers of personal budget holders, the approach is not significantly changing their services or improving their quality of life.

Investing in support services

Evidence from personal budgets highlights the importance of information, advice and support in enabling people to fully understand the different available options, to make best use of a personal budget and in encouraging the take-up of direct payments. This is especially the case for older people and people with mental health problems where take-up has generally lagged behind. Research by the National Audit Office (2011) found that a significant proportion of personal budget holders found choosing and purchasing care and support difficult. However, the proportion of personal budget holders offered help to plan their support by their local authority ranged from just over a third to more than four fifths. Budget holders themselves prefer support services that are provided by user-led or disabled people's organisations or support from peers who have direct experience of using a personal budget. In social care, these types of support have also been found to be more likely to lead to more budget holders opting for direct payments (Campbell et al, 2011).

The successful roll-out of PHBs will equally depend on investment in the infrastructure to provide information, advice and support to PHB holders. This is discussed in greater detail in Section 2. Much of this can be developed in partnership with local authorities and existing user-led and peer support services.

Limit the bureaucracy of personalisation

In its 2011 assessment of progress made in implementing *Putting People First*, the national partnership for the delivery of personalisation in social care, Think Local Act Personal, highlighted the need to tackle bureaucracy as a major challenge in moving forward. The growth in bureaucracy was commonly found to be linked to the following:

- the lack of a single point of contact for individuals to seek support;
- the development of overly complex resource allocation systems that require long development timescales;
- confusion over the level of information required in a support plan before resources can be released;
- the imposition of restrictive menus of services and complicated rules about how personal budgets can be used;
- a disproportionate approach to monitoring how resources are used rather than a focus on whether or not outcomes are achieved (Routledge and Lewis, 2011).

The bureaucracy associated with personal budgets affects all parties in the process. Budget holders experience delays and frustrations in securing approval for their support plans that can erode their satisfaction. Professionals find that they are under greater work pressure and face additional hurdles in securing services for individuals, and administrators have to deal with more complex business processes. Overall, growth in bureaucracy makes it less likely that personal budgets will improve cost-effectiveness.

Experience from the PHB pilot highlights significant variation in how PHBs were implemented, with some areas adopting more bureaucratic approaches to decision making than others (Davidson et al, 2012). For example, some pilot sites relied on panels to approve care plans, while others relied on decision making by a single clinician. Experience from social care confirms the findings of the national PHB evaluation that streamlining the PHB process and maintaining flexibility will be critical to sustaining support for personalisation as well as maximising the potential of PHBs to improve individual health and wellbeing and value for money.

Investing in culture change

One of the criticisms levelled against personal budgets is that, in many local authorities, their roll-out has not been supported by wider culture change in adult social care. As a result, personal budgets have become a new delivery mechanism for social care services and supports rather than the catalyst for changing the relationships between disabled people, those who support them and the wider welfare state. As we saw earlier,

Putting People First did identify wider changes that needed to accompany personal budgets, but with demanding targets to meet, these broader aspects of culture change often got lost (SCIE and nef, 2011).

According to a former president of the Association of Directors of Adult Social Services (ADASS), there are two areas of cultural change that are essential if personal budgets are to succeed in achieving a better life for disabled people. The first is to see those who need support as genuine partners rather than passive recipients of services – individuals with assets and talents who can play an equal role alongside professionals in identifying their goals and designing how those goals can best be met. The second is to move away from thinking about social care as a set of services and to redefine the purpose of good support as being to reconnect people to their communities, to help them rebuild meaningful roles in society and to support citizenship. This means greater use of peer support, user-led organisations, community-based activities and universal services over specialist, commissioned services (Jones, 2012).

These changes in social care have much in common with the culture change that PHBs seek to bring about in the NHS by recognising individual expertise, addressing health in the context of a person's wider needs and focusing on inclusion in society, not just access to services. In many ways, this is even tougher to achieve in the NHS because it is a more medicalised and more professionally driven system. Ensuring that there is a sound understanding of the culture change that PHBs necessitate and adequate investment in training will be essential to the success of national roll-out.

Developing a national approach

Despite a binding target on local authorities for the implementation of personal budgets up until 2011 and ongoing national commitments, there is significant variation in take-up rates across local authorities and across different disability groups. This means that an individual's experience of personalisation in social care will be very different depending on where they live.

Social care has always tolerated variation. The application of Fair Access to Care Services (FACS) criteria that determine eligibility for council-funded social care has always been done locally. While variation undeniably exists in the NHS, a postcode lottery in health raises more criticism given the universal nature of the NHS. This poses a question about the roll-out of PHBs. Without a national target and with clinical commissioning groups (CCGs) driving the process, the experience from social care suggests that access to PHBs is likely to vary dramatically from one area to the next. Not only will the value of a PHB be different in each area, but the availability of PHBs for particular conditions is also likely to vary. It remains to be seen whether the public will tolerate this.

The next chapter looks in greater depth at the contribution that PHBs can make to the management of long-term conditions that account for the bulk of spending in today's NHS. The chapter highlights how PHBs are part of a family of initiatives that are seeking to drive the take-up of shared decision making in the NHS. However, in many important ways, PHBs are different from other approaches, and it is these differences that underpin their potential to make a unique contribution to the lives of those with long-term health conditions and disabilities.

FOUR

Managing long-term conditions: the case for personal health budgets

As we saw earlier, the majority of spending in the NHS is on long-term conditions such as diabetes, arthritis, COPD and depression that cannot be cured but have to be managed on a day-to-day basis. Figure 4.1 shows the proportion of people in England who report having a long-term condition at different ages, and highlights how the proportion living with a long-term condition increases with age, with older people typically living with more than one condition. Up to 80 per cent of GP consultations in England are with people with long-term conditions, and the 15 per cent of people with three or more long-term conditions account for almost 30 per cent of inpatient days in hospitals (Wilson, 2005).

Figure 4.1: The proportion of people with long-term conditions by age in England

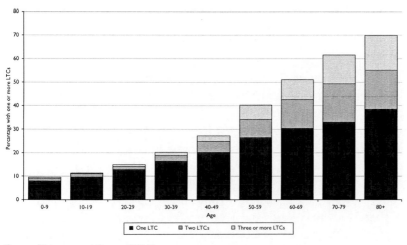

Source: Alakeson and Rosen (2011)

Much of the cost of long-term conditions stems from avoidable hospitalisations when day-to-day management at home breaks down. Effective management of long-term conditions falls more to individuals and their families than to healthcare professionals. If there are 8,760 hours in a year, the average person with a long-term condition in the UK spends no more than three or four hours a year with a health professional (Hannan, 2010). Even someone receiving intensive treatment, for example, from an assertive outreach team for a serious mental health problem, would see that team for no more than three hours a week – less than 2 per cent of the hours in the year (Alakeson and Perkins, 2012).

The evidence base for the positive impact of individual engagement in the management of long-term conditions is strong. Research has demonstrated that enabling patients to actively participate in all aspects of their care, such as choices about treatment and self-management, results in better adherence to medications and improved management of long-term conditions without increasing costs (Hibbard et al, 2004). There is evidence of less use of hospital services (Gibson et al, 2004; Newman et al, 2004) and better outcomes associated with support for self-care (Lorig et al, 1999). Patient engagement contributes to patient safety by ensuring that patients' behaviour, choices and needs are accurately communicated to clinical professionals, and it reduces anxiety and depression for individuals and improves their ability to cope with adversity (Epstein et al, 2010). This has led to recognition of the importance of patient engagement as part of any model of effective care management (Wagner, 1998).

Yet surveys have shown that many patients are not supported by clinicians to manage their condition day to day. Figure 4.2 shows the percentage of primary care doctors in 11 countries who report routinely giving patients with long-term conditions written instructions about how to manage their care at home. At a third of all GPs, the NHS is a high performer by international standards, but a third is still inadequate to deal with the growing burden of long-term conditions. Even when information is provided to individuals, they do not always understand it (RCP, 2012). According to a survey of people with long-term conditions in the UK, over 90 per cent are interested in being more active self-carers and over 75 per cent would feel more confident about this if they had help from a healthcare professional or peer. But 30 per cent have never been encouraged by a professional to take control of their own care (DH, 2005). The failure of clinical staff to provide active support for patient engagement has been identified as the most significant barrier to increasing engagement (Richards and Coulter, 2007).

Figure 4.2: Percentage of primary care physicians saying they routinely give chronically ill patients written instructions on managing care at home

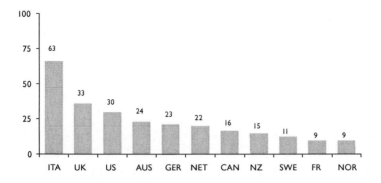

Source: Commonwealth Fund International Survey (2009) (www.commonwealthfund.org/Content/Publications/In-the-Literature/2009/Nov/A-Survey-of-Primary-Care-Physicians.aspx)

Shared decision making in health

Given the centrality of individual engagement to the effective management of long-term conditions, there has been a growth in recent years of initiatives that are rooted in the concept of shared decision making. Shared decision making takes as its starting point the fact that there are very few areas of healthcare where there is only one treatment option. In the vast majority of cases, there are several possibilities, each with different risks, side-effects and likelihood of success. Shared decision making therefore seeks to bring together clinical evidence with the informed preferences of individuals. It can apply to any aspect of care where the situation is not immediately life-threatening and the patient has the mental capacity to make a decision. This includes decisions about tests, treatment options and the ongoing management of conditions. The defining features of shared decision making are as follows:

- Patients and clinicians act collaboratively to make decisions, each recognising the (differing) expertise of the other. Decisions are based on both clinical evidence and the patient's informed preferences.
- Patients and clinicians have reliable, accessible, evidence-based information to inform decision making that explains care and treatment options, potential outcomes, risks and uncertainties. An individual's lifestyle, needs, preferences, aspirations and attitudes to

risk are also recognised as important factors in the decision-making process.

- Clinicians ensure that patients have effective support to make an informed decision through conversations with a clinician or health coach and access to decision aids such as leaflets, DVDs, websites and interactive computer programs.
- Decisions are systematically recorded and implemented, and communicated to all who need to be involved, patients as well as clinicians (Edwards and Elwyn, 2009).

Shared decision making has been shown to result in happier, less anxious patients but also to produce decisions that are more in keeping with patients' preferences and supported by clinical evidence. If patients make decisions with their doctor, they are much more likely to defer treatment or opt for no treatment than their doctor, with no measurable adverse impact on health outcomes or satisfaction (Coulter and Collins, 2011). However, despite this strong evidence base, adoption into clinical practice has been slow. Recent initiatives such as the Expert Patient Programme (Rogers et al, 2006), Year of Care (2011), Co-creating Health (Wallace et al, 2012) and People-powered Health (Horne et al, 2013) are all rooted in the philosophy of shared decision making and have sought to change practice in line with its principles. Table 4.1 identifies the core features of each initiative. As discussed in Chapter 1, a focus on partnership is also one of the central features of PHBs, and PHBs can be seen as part of this same family of initiatives. However, as we discuss later in this chapter, while the initiatives have important similarities, the differences between them are critical to understanding where one approach is better suited than another.

Similarities and differences

At the centre of all of the initiatives in Table 4.1 and central also to PHBs is the care planning process. More often than not, care plans for long-term conditions are static documents into which individuals have little input. They are completed by professionals rather than being owned by individuals. For example, a significant motivation for the Year of Care programme was the gap between the high proportion of patients who had an annual review for the management of their diabetes and the much smaller number who reported discussing their goals and treatment options with their doctor (Year of Care, 2011). Instead of being a one-off event, care planning as described here is intended to be an ongoing, collaborative process that underpins the partnership between individuals and professionals. Section 2 discusses how this approach to care planning can be implemented in the context of PHBs.

In addition to care planning, to make a reality of partnership, each of the initiatives described in Table 4.1 requires a common set of building blocks that are also important for PHBs. They include: access to information and decision support tools for individuals; training for health professionals in motivational interviewing and other forms of non-directed communication; and the development of information technology systems to record and retrieve care planning decisions. Each initiative also faces a similar set of barriers to widespread adoption, the biggest being the need for culture change within the NHS. Clinical professionals are trained to manage risk on behalf of individuals and take decisions based on scientific evidence. Shared decision-making initiatives involve sharing risk and the pros and cons of different options with individuals as part of working in partnership.

Alongside these similarities, there are five important areas of difference between the shared decision-making initiatives described in Table 4.1 and PHBs. First is the scope of the partnership between individuals and professionals, with PHBs adopting a broad conception of health and wellbeing, while most of the other initiatives remain more focused on treatment decisions. Second, PHBs take a whole person approach, while other initiatives such as Year of Care are condition-specific. This means that the Year of Care will deal with an individual's diabetes care and any related goals, while a PHB would look at an individual's needs and desired outcomes more holistically. Third, PHBs look far beyond health interventions to focus on any good or service or other community resource that an individual feels will benefit their care. The other initiatives are more focused on healthcare interventions, although People-powered Heath also recognises the need to commission other services to complement clinical care. This relates to the fourth area of difference, that is the nature of evidence. Co-creating Health and Year of Care continue to adopt a traditional view of evidence-based care that is rooted in clinical evidence, while PHBs place greater value on personal views of whether or not a particular approach appears to work for an individual. Finally, as discussed in Chapter 1, PHBs are the only initiative described here that involve a transfer of power from the professional to the individual through the allocation of money to the budget holder. This potentially puts the collaboration between the professional and individual on a stronger footing.

Table 4.1: Shared decision-making initiatives in the NHS

Initiative	Objective	Content	Evidence/findings
National Expert Patient Programme (2002–ongoing)	To allow people with long-term conditions to take control of their health and better manage their condition on a daily basis	Six group sessions led by trained lay people who live with one or more long-term conditions. Sessions focus on self-care issues commonly faced by individuals living with an ongoing health condition, such as communicating with family and professionals and dealing with pain and tiredness	A randomised controlled trial found the programme to be moderately effective in improving self-efficacy and energy levels in people with long-term conditions. It was also found to be cost-effective because an overall reduction in service utilisation offset the cost of the intervention
Year of Care (2007–ongoing) Initial pilot project took place in Tower Hamlets PCT, Calderdale and Kirklees PCTs and North Tyneside and West Northumberland PCTs	To improve the care of people with diabetes. Now extended to COPD and to long-term conditions more broadly	Year of Care involves personalised care planning supported by a more collaborative relationship with the individual's clinician and effective local commissioning. To improve care planning, Year of Care introduced a two-step process, involving an information-gathering session with a healthcare assistant followed by a review with a GP to develop an action plan	Effective care planning consultations were found to rely on three elements: an engaged, empowered patient; healthcare professionals committed to a partnership approach; and appropriate, robust organisational systems. Each element is important and interdependent. If one element is weak or missing the service is not fit for purpose

Table 4.1: continued

Initiative	Objective	Content	Evidence/findings
Co-creating Health demonstration programme (2007-12)	To enable people with a long-term condition to 'improve their health and have a better quality of life by taking a more active role in their own care'. Sites focused on COPD, depression, diabetes or musculoskeletal pain in a mix of primary and secondary settings	The programme consists of two modules: the Self-Management Programme (SMP) for people with long-term conditions and the Advanced Development Programme (ADP) for clinicians. Both programmes were spread over a number of sessions and co-facilitated by a person who was successfully managing their long-term condition and a clinician. Both programmes focused on three enablers: goal setting; shared agenda setting; and goal follow-up	The 882 participants in the SMP reported statistically significant changes in positive engagement in life, adopting a more constructive attitude and approach to their condition and enjoying more positive emotional wellbeing. The 437 clinicians in the ADP reported increased motivation to improve their practice and greater belief that improvement was possible, increased job satisfaction, and a greater sense that they were now 'helping people' in a way that reflected why they came into healthcare
People-powered Health programme run in six areas from 2011-13: Calderdale, Earl's Court, Lambeth, Leeds, Newcastle and Stockport	Makes the case for changing the ways in which healthcare is organised to better combine the very best scientific and clinical knowledge with the expertise and commitment of patients themselves	Nesta and the Innovation Unit supported local teams in six areas to work on an aspect of service redesign that fitted with the overall vision of People-powered Health, that is, a healthcare system that recognises individual assets, is built on a partnership between individuals and professionals and puts the individual at the centre of the healthcare delivery system	The programme identified three critical changes required to support a people-powered healthcare system: changing consultations to be structured conversations; commissioning new services to complement clinical care; and co-designing pathways for long-term conditions

Source: Alakeson et al (2013)

Figure 4.3 illustrates how each of the initiatives relates to the other as a family rooted in shared decision making. The scope of the partnership, from single condition to whole person, sits on the vertical axis and the scope of the solution, from healthcare interventions to any possible solution, on the horizontal axis. This puts PHBs in the top right-hand corner of Figure 4.3, responding to the needs of the whole person and drawing on resources from any service or community organisation. People-powered Health sits close to it. Diagonally opposite, in the bottom left-hand corner, are more traditional initiatives such as Co-creating Health that focus on a partnership to address a single condition, with solutions confined to evidence-based, healthcare interventions.

Figure 4.3: The relationship between shared decision-making initiatives

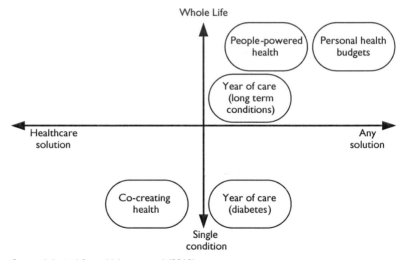

Source: Adapted from Alakeson et al (2013)

From shared decision making to co-production

In part the different orientation of PHBs from other shared decision-making initiatives stems from the fact that PHBs also draw heavily on the concept of 'co-production'. Co-production recognises that positive social outcomes can only be created if those who provide services work together with those who use services:

> Services do not produce social outcomes; people do.
> Recycling happens because of the people involved.

Householders separate waste, compost some of it at home and put the rest out for their local council services to collect and recycle. The police and the courts could not apprehend and prosecute criminals were it not for members of the public; it is they who are the major detectors of crimes. Schools provide education but it is parents who support their children's learning. In each case, what we are seeing is social outcomes – a sustainable environment, community safety and educational attainment – being co-produced through the joint efforts of service users and services. (Cummins and Miller, 2007 , p 1)

The acceptance of the logic of co-production leads to a focus on the beneficiaries of services as assets whose capabilities can be harnessed to improve social outcomes. Co-production emphasises the development of connections between people to bring about change rather than the provision of services, and seeks to create opportunities for self-help and reciprocity. Finally, it shifts the role of the state and service providers from doing things for people to enabling them to act for themselves in pursuit of their own goals. Co-production demands a more radical rethink of the role of the NHS and other public services than shared decision making, and some of the dimensions of PHBs such as their whole person orientation and focus on social inclusion draw particularly on this strand of thinking (Horne et al, 2013).

The six principles of co-production in public services

1. Recognising people as assets (rather than problems).
2. Building on people's capabilities (rather than just focusing on their needs).
3. Mutuality and reciprocity (rather than passive consumption of public services).
4. Peer support networks (that complement bilateral relationships between professionals and service users).
5. Blurring distinctions between producers and consumers (with service users being actively involved in producing outcomes).
6. Facilitating rather than just delivering services.

Source: Boyle et al (2010).

The different orientation of PHBs from other shared decision-making initiatives allows them to make a unique contribution to the management of long-term conditions. The national pilot programme has enabled significant experimentation with the use of PHBs for a range of long-term conditions and has helped to identify several areas where they can add particular value:

- PHBs allow individuals to tailor care exactly to their needs and preferences and can, thereby, maximise individual engagement. Other initiatives such as Year of Care have worked closely with third sector organisations to commission alternatives to NHS self-management supports, but are less able to respond to specific individual needs.
- By allowing individuals to go outside of commissioned services, PHBs can effectively meet the needs of those for whom the standard NHS offer is not appropriate. The pilot programme revealed that the standard NHS offer for physiotherapy, counselling and similar therapies of six to eight weeks at a time of acute need does not work well for everyone. Some people need ongoing, maintenance therapy or therapy when they require it. These individuals' needs can be better met in the private sector, as Yve's experience with PHBs illustrates (see page 83).
- By their very nature, long-term conditions affect day-to-day life and the important roles that people value such as being a parent or going to work. The whole person scope of PHBs and their focus on solutions beyond healthcare make them uniquely responsive to this wider aspect of the effective management of long-term conditions. For those with multiple long-term conditions, PHBs provide a tool that can look beyond the needs of any one condition to address the whole person in the context of their family and wider social situation.

This chapter has highlighted the importance of individual engagement in the effective management of long-term conditions and described a family of initiatives that seek to make individuals more equal partners in their care. PHBs are part of this shift and this chapter makes the case for them as an important new tool for the management of long-term conditions. However, their role is not exclusive. Each initiative described in this chapter has a part to play in the care each of us may need. For example, an individual with diabetes may be part of the diabetes Year of Care programme through which he develops a care plan with his doctor. A small part of that care plan may be delivered in the form of a PHB to allow him to better manage his diet and exercise. Alongside this, he may choose to access the Expert Patient Programme run by his local NHS trust. If his condition becomes unstable and he finds himself in hospital, he would hope that the clinical team at the hospital will use the principles of shared decision making to ensure that he is fully informed and engaged in treatment decisions.

The next chapter turns to current evidence of the impact of PHBs on the management of long-term conditions, looking at individual engagement, satisfaction with services, quality of life, health outcomes and costs. It draws on UK and international studies from health and social care. The chapter starts with a discussion of the nature of evidence in healthcare and the implications for PHBs.

FIVE

How well do personal health budgets work?

The question of what constitutes evidence is not a straightforward one. In healthcare, a hierarchy of evidence has tended to operate which sets systematic reviews and randomised controlled trials (RCTs) as the gold standard, as illustrated in Table 5.1. A controlled study or trial compares outcomes for two groups: a treatment group that gets the intervention and a control group that does not. An RCT assigns individuals to one group or the other on a random basis and thereby tries to eliminate any biases within the two groups to isolate the impact of the intervention. The reliance on controlled studies in healthcare reflects the dominance of drug trials that are usually RCTs in shaping notions of evidence, and has been accelerated by the work of the National Institute for Health and Clinical Excellence (NICE) on evidence-based care.

Table 5.1: A hierarchy of evidence

Hierarchy	Type of evidence
Type I	At least one good systemic review, including at least one randomised controlled trial
Type II	At least one good randomised controlled trial
Type III	At least one well-designed intervention study without randomisation
Type IV	At least one well-designed observational study
Type V	Expert opinion, including the views of service users and carers

Source: DH (1999, p 6)

However, questions are now being raised about the applicability of RCTs to evaluations of healthcare interventions and the dominance of this form of evidence (Cesar et al, 2004). First, it can take many years for the findings from an RCT study to be reported. This can slow down the rate of adoption of the intervention and, even when the results are positive, there is no guarantee that the intervention will be implemented in day-to-day practice (Steventon, 2012). Second, many clinical procedures and pharmaceuticals are recommended within clinical practice on the basis that they work for 50 per cent of people in the trial. This means that they do not work for the other

50 per cent. The incomplete nature of the clinical evidence base to inform decisions about care for any one specific individual highlights the need for other forms of evidence to fill in the gaps and is discussed further in Section 3 (Hasnain-Wynia, 2006). Third, certain academics have challenged the very existence of a hierarchy of evidence, arguing that different types of evidence are required to assess the impact of health interventions because each assesses different dimensions and can add value to the overall picture. For example, a controlled evaluation may be most appropriate when looking at clinical effectiveness, but patient interviews may be better placed to tell you whether or not the experience of the intervention was positive (Glasby et al, 2007; Glasby, 2011a).

In the context of PHBs and self-direction in healthcare internationally, reliance on the gold standard of RCTs poses particular problems. For practical reasons, it is necessary to draw on a wider range of evidence. Self-direction is new to healthcare and the English PHB pilot is by far the most comprehensive experiment of its kind in the world. There is relatively little evidence from controlled studies to draw on outside of the national evaluation and on which this chapter draws heavily (Forder et al, 2012).

The personal health budgets evaluation

The PHB evaluation (www.phbe.org.uk) used a controlled trial to compare the experiences of just over 1,000 people selected to receive a PHB with those of just over 1,000 continuing with conventional support arrangements across six conditions: COPD, diabetes, long-term neurological conditions, mental health, stroke and patients eligible for NHS CHC. In some of the 20 evaluation sites, people were randomised into the PHB or control group. In others, the PHB group was recruited from the caseloads of professionals offering PHBs and the control group from non-participating healthcare professionals. The evaluation followed a mixed design, using both quantitative and qualitative methodologies to explore patient outcomes, experiences, service use and costs.

Main findings:

- The use of PHBs was associated with a significant improvement in the care-related quality of life and psychological wellbeing of patients.
- PHBs did not have an impact on health status or on clinical measures over a 12-month follow-up period. But equally there was no evidence of deterioration in health when individuals were given control of their care.
- PHBs had a more positive effect if they were implemented with flexibility over what could be purchased and how the budget could be managed.

- There were no significant differences in outcomes by age, sex or socio-economic status.
- PHBs were found to reduce the costs of inpatient care compared to the control group.
- PHBs were found to be more cost-effective using care-related quality of life than conventional service delivery.
- In particular, PHBs were found to be cost-effective for CHC, mental health, for larger PHBs over £1,000 and for PHBs that were implemented in keeping with the ethos of the policy of greater choice and control for individuals.

Intellectually, given that a central purpose of PHBs is to create a patient–centred NHS and to support people to meet their own health and wellbeing objectives, a broader range of evidence from all levels of the hierarchy in Table 5.1 is required to assess their success. To judge whether PHB holders feel empowered and value the experience is probably best ascertained by talking to them, even if this type of evidence sits at the bottom of the hierarchy.

For these reasons, this chapter deliberately draws on a broad range of evidence to identify what is known about the impact of PHBs so far. The chapter focuses on evidence related to self-directed initiatives that are primarily health–related rather than social care. However, given limited evidence related specifically to health and a greater number of controlled studies of self-direction in social care, the chapter does draw on evidence from social care where relevant, although it does not present a complete overview of the evidence for personalisation in social care. The chapter incorporates as much evidence as possible from international studies. This raises a particular challenge when it comes to differentiating between health and social care. Each country draws the dividing line between the two systems in a different place and, therefore, programmes that would be similar to PHBs sit formally within the social care system (Alakeson, 2010). The Dutch *persoonsgedonden budget* (PGB) is a good example. PGBs are part of the long–term care insurance system rather than the health insurance system. However, PGBs are discussed in this chapter because they share many similarities with PHBs in CHC (White, 2011). Outside of PHBs, the main programmes and pilots that are discussed in this chapter are described in Table 5.2.

Table 5.2: International initiatives in self-directed care

Initiative	Population	Evaluation
Cash & Counseling demonstration (USA) www.bc.edu/schools/gssw/ nrcpds/cash_and_counseling.html	Three-state Medicaid demonstration to give individuals with long-term care needs receiving personal assistance and other home and community-based services control of their services and supports. The demonstration included adults with physical and learning disabilities, children with significant health needs and older adults	RCT evaluation using quantitative and qualitative methods, with a three-year follow-up in one state
Individual budget pilot (UK) http://php.york.ac.uk/inst/spru/ research/summs/ibsen.php	Two-year pilot in 13 local authorities to offer disabled adults and older people an integrated individual budget across six funding streams that provide support for disabilities	RCT evaluation using quantitative and qualitative methods
Consumer Directed Care initiative (Australia) www.health.gov.au/cdc	Two-year initiative to support 1,000 individuals receiving community aged care and 400 carers to make informed choices about the types of services they received, how they were delivered and by whom	Mixed methods evaluation using non-matched treatment and control groups
Persoonsgedonden budget (PGB) (The Netherlands)	PGBs introduced in 1996 for people with long-term care needs not covered by the health insurance system. PGBs cover personal care, nursing care, support services, such as day care, and short stays away from home, including respite care	User surveys and other qualitative evaluation
Pflegebudgets (personal budgets) demonstration for long-term care services and supports (Germany)	Demonstration comparing care outcomes and costs of *Pflegebudgets* with traditional long-term agency care and existing cash payments for care in seven counties between 2004 and 2008	RCT evaluation using quantitative and qualitative methods
Consumer Recovery Investment Funds (CRIF) – Self-directed Care (USA)	Two-year pilot in Delaware County, Pennsylvania, to give individuals with serious mental health problems choice and control over their outpatient behavioural health services within a managed care context	RCT evaluation being undertaken by Temple University, Philadelphia

Table 5.2: continued

Initiative	Population	Evaluation
Florida Self-directed Care (USA) www.flsdc.org	Programme established in 2000 for individuals with serious mental health problems to control their own services and supports. It operates in the Jacksonville and Fort Myers areas of the state and is run by the Florida Department of Children and Families	Pre- and post-evaluation and regular analysis of administrative data conducted by Florida legislature
Empowerment Initiatives, Oregon (USA) www.chooseempowerment.com	Peer-run brokerage including a non-recurring individual budget to support people with serious mental health problems towards recovery over a two-year period. In one county the brokerage is focused on supporting people to move from group homes to independent living	User surveys and qualitative evaluation
Texas Self-directed Care (USA) www.texassdc.org	Two-year pilot programme operated by the North Texas Behavioral Health Authority in its seven county area to give individuals with serious mental health problems choice and control over their outpatient behavioural health services within a managed care context	RCT evaluation being undertaken by the University of Illinois, Chicago

This chapter discusses the available evidence for PHBs within the following categories:

• evidence related to patient-centred care
• evidence related to healthcare quality and service use
• evidence related to health and other outcomes
• evidence related to cost-effectiveness.

Patient-centred care

As discussed in the Introduction to this book, patient-centredness is increasingly recognised as an important dimension of high quality healthcare, if not the principle measure of quality, as Don Berwick has suggested (Berwick, 2009b). On this dimension, the evidence is strong. International studies consistently report positive impacts for budget holders (Health Foundation, 2010). For example, interviews with 52 PHB holders participating in the national pilot in England found that the majority reported positive impacts nine months after they first received a PHB, with a few respondents describing PHBs as 'life changing'. Just under a fifth felt that their PHB had had no impact and only one person reported negative consequences, although implementation issues can account for most of the reported dissatisfaction (Davidson et al, 2012, p 5). Similarly, among 31 participants in the Texas Self-directed Care pilot, 90 per cent rated the programme 'excellent' or 'good' and only 10 per cent 'fair'. No participants rated the programme as 'poor' (Norris et al, 2010). Equally positive views have been found in surveys of social care (Hatton and Waters, 2011).

These overall positive views incorporate different dimensions of patient–centredness, each of which is important. The first is that self-direction, as intended, has been shown to provide individuals with greater choice and control than traditional healthcare delivery in specifying their needs, in the types of services and supports they can use and in the flexibility they have to manage their budget (Gordon et al, 2012). The final report of the national PHB evaluation attributes much of the improvement in quality of life and wellbeing to this increase in control, stating that 'the benefits ... appear to stem from the value people place on increased choice and control in their lives, and the capability this brings for people to improve the more complex or higher-order aspects of their quality of life' (Forder et al, 2012, p 79).

The flexibility of self-direction is apparent in the purchases that individuals with similar conditions make to improve their health and wellbeing. Table 5.3 shows the range of goods and services purchased in the Florida Self-directed Care program. While individuals are careful to ensure their mental health condition is well managed and continue to purchase clinical services such as counselling and medication management, they also pursue their wellbeing through a diverse range of non–traditional routes, much as we saw in the purchases made in the PHB pilot reported in Table 2.1.

A second important dimension of patient–centredness is that self-direction has been shown to address health in a holistic way that better reflects individuals' views than the organisational structures of traditional healthcare delivery. For example, some of the early requests from participants in both the Texas Self-directed Care pilot and the Consumer Recovery Investment Funds (CRIF) pilot were to address physical health needs such as eye and foot problems despite the fact that their eligibility for the pilot was based on their mental health needs (Maule, 2010; Norris et al, 2010). Among participants in Texas

Table 5.3: Purchases made by participants in the Florida Self-directed Care program in the Fort Myers area in the first six months of the fiscal year 2009–10

Type of purchase	Cash value ($)	Percentage of total spending
Transportation	10,940	13
Computers and accessories	10,029	12
Dental services	9,684	11
Medication management services	7,119	8
Psychotropic medications	7,107	8
Mental health counselling	7,069	8
Housing	6,009	7
Massage, weight control, smoking cessation	4,386	5
Utilities	2,862	3
Travel	2,502	3
Equipment	2,349	3
Clothing	2,069	2
Food	2,021	2
Crafts	1,979	2
Licences/certification	1,822	2
Entertainment (movies, eating out, etc)	1,768	2
Vision services	1,639	2
Furniture	931	1
Non-mental health medical	749	1
Camera and supplies	694	1
Education, training and materials	573	1
Hair cut, manicure, make-up lessons	489	1
Pet ownership	481	1
Supplies and storage	410	<1
Other	12	<1
Total	**85,693**	**100**

Source: OPPAGA (2010)

Self-directed Care, 55 per cent reported better physical health since joining the pilot. The PHB evaluation in England reported similar findings, with those receiving a PHB for a physical health condition reporting improvements in their mental health and vice versa (Davidson et al, 2012, p 22).

Third, self-direction has been shown to improve access to services. This was an important finding from the Cash & Counseling demonstration in the US that remains one of the largest and most rigorous international studies of self-direction in social care. It found that those who were directing their own services were more likely to get the amount of care to which they were entitled compared to those who were receiving services from a care agency through the traditional model (Dale et al, 2004). A similar finding was reported in the *Pflegebudgets* demonstration in Germany. Personal budget recipients received 37 per cent more hours of care than those using agency services (Artnz and Thomsen, 2008). In the Netherlands, the explosion of PGBs from 5,401 in 1996 to 123,000 in 2010 in large part reflects an increase in take-up among parents of children with autism and attention deficit hyperactivity disorder (ADHD) for whom the traditional system was not able to provide any appropriate services. Although the influx of people into PGBs has created sustainability issues for the system (discussed later in this chapter), families are undeniably getting better access to services than they would otherwise (White, 2011).

The national evaluation of PHBs in England found that around half of the PHB holders interviewed were incurring additional private costs for health-related items for which the NHS would not pay but which they felt were beneficial, including acupuncture, physiotherapy, counselling and gym memberships. Around half of those interviewed were unhappy that the traditional NHS did not cover these treatments and were worried about the long-term costs of paying for them out of their own pocket. Some saw a PHB as a way of meeting these costs (Irvine et al, 2011). Similarly, a survey of nearly 500 people with musculoskeletal conditions conducted by Arthritis Research UK found that 74 per cent of respondents had spent their own money on interventions which they felt contributed positively to their health over the previous 12 months, including diet and nutrition supplements, massage and equipment to help with daily tasks such as bathing or getting around (Arthritis Research UK, 2012).

As well as creating more patient-centred care, the PHB evaluation indicates that carers and other family members also report positive views, although there is not necessarily a corresponding reduction in the use of informal care (Davidson et al, 2012; Forder et al, 2012). This echoes findings from personal budgets in social care (Tyson et al, 2010). These positive views appear to stem from carers of PHB holders reporting a better quality of life and better perceived health than carers of non-PHB holders, as well as the knowledge that their loved ones are receiving more appropriate care and, therefore, also enjoy a better quality of life.

Service use and quality

While there are generally concerns that PHBs will erode the quality of healthcare by allowing individuals to purchase services that do not have a sound evidence base according to the hierarchy of evidence in Table 5.1 (Mathers et al, 2012), qualitative studies of budget holders indicate the opposite: quality improves with control. For example, 74 per cent of participants in the Texas Self-directed Care pilot reported that the services they were buying themselves were better than those they had previously received through the traditional Medicaid mental health system. Only 7 per cent said the services were worse (Norris et al, 2010). Participants in a similar programme in Oregon gave self-directed care a higher rating across the board than the traditional system. They felt that self-directed services involved them more, were more culturally sensitive and gave them more of the information and education they needed to reach their recovery goals (Sullivan, 2006). The individual budget pilot found that younger people with physical disabilities reported higher quality of care and were more satisfied with the help they received (Glendinning et al, 2008).

These possibly surprising findings related to quality highlight differences in how the healthcare system judges quality compared to individuals. The system places greater emphasis on formal qualifications and training and on the existence of documented procedures for certain aspects of care and is less focused on the day-to-day experience of care by individuals and families. Therefore, services that meet standards in theory are often poor quality in practice. As a Dutch provider of support for PGB holders commented, 'qualifications don't necessarily translate into good care. How do you recognise quality when there is no evidence base? Quality is help that works. And if it doesn't work, it's your [the budget holder's] responsibility to sort it out' (White, 2011, p 17).

One of the major dissatisfactions with traditional NHS services expressed by PHB holders in the national evaluation in England was the unreliability and inflexibility of care agencies (Davidson et al, 2012). Although care agencies have to meet standards determined by the Care Quality Commission (CQC) to win NHS contracts, interviews with PHB holders demonstrate several ways in which PHBs improve on the quality provided by traditional agencies.

First, agencies cannot guarantee continuity of care and often send a different carer each day, which means that carers do not accumulate knowledge and expertise about the individual and family with whom they are working. This is a particular challenge for those with high levels of need or who cannot communicate verbally. By hiring their own care teams, PHB holders can improve their continuity of care, particularly if they can set their own pay rates and create incentives for workers to stay with them for longer. International studies have highlighted that from a family perspective, the core of good care is weighted towards knowing the individual and family rather than having specific formal qualifications, with many families not hiring on the basis of formal training or criminal background checks (Doty and O'Keeffe, 2010).

Second, families report that the care they receive from their own care teams is more reliable than agency care. A similar finding was reported by PHB holders in the *Pfelgebudget* demonstration in Germany (Arntz and Thomsen, 2008a). In large part, greater reliability goes hand in hand with continuity. The relationship between the PHB holder and the team makes both parties less likely to let the other down. Families can also plan for contingencies more effectively with their own staff to ensure cover for holidays or sick days because the staff work as a team in contrast to agency staff who tend to work for more than one family. These aspects of quality are well illustrated by Stephen's experience (see page vi) of using a PHB instead of the care agency sent by his PCT to meet his continuing healthcare needs. The issue of quality is discussed further in Section 3.

Looking at service use, the PHB evaluation shows that PHB holders make less use of inpatient care than those receiving traditional services, suggesting that PHBs support prevention and health maintenance (Forder et al, 2012). For example, as we saw in Chapter 1 with Malcolm who has dementia, his PHB has allowed him to significantly reduce his medication and he no longer receives any clinical input from specialist services. Similar examples have been reported in other pilot sites. A young man with mental health problems was able to avoid an inpatient admission by using a laptop he had purchased with a small, one-off PHB. The laptop enabled him to stay in contact with his early intervention team, avoiding the need for an admission (Coyle, 2009).

These findings from the PHB evaluation that show lower service use are supported by a small number of international studies. A study of participants in the Florida Self-directed Care program found that those directing their own care were less likely to use crisis services and more likely to use routine services than those in the traditional system, although the two groups were not matched (Florida Department of Children and Families, 2007). Participants in the Cash & Counseling demonstration in Arkansas made 18 per cent less use of nursing home services over a three-year follow-up period than those in the control group who received traditional Medicaid services (Dale and Brown, 2006).

Health and other outcomes

Several programmes and pilots have demonstrated improvements in self-reported health. For example, the majority of PHB holders interviewed for the national evaluation in England said that their PHB had had a positive impact on their health, including reductions in pain, better pain management, improvements in mobility and improvements in general health and wellbeing (Davidson et al, 2012). These findings build on evidence from social care in which individuals report health improvements from having control of their social care services through a personal budget (Tyson et al, 2010). This highlights the significance of the process of taking control discussed earlier.

Going beyond self-reported measures, there are only a small number of studies that report improvements in health outcomes (Gadsby, 201). One study of 106 participants in the Florida Self-directed Care program found that participants scored significantly higher on the Global Assessment of Functioning Scale in the year after enrolment compared to the year prior to enrolment. However, the study is based on an assessment of the participants before and after the programme with no control group and is, therefore, not highly reliable by academic standards (Cook et al, 2008). Turning again to evidence from social care, there is reliable evidence from the Cash & Counseling evaluation that individuals who controlled their own personal care services saw improvements in their health outcomes. Older adults in the New Jersey demonstration were significantly less likely to fall or to develop contractures or have contractures worsen than the control group, and working-age adults were significantly less likely to fall. Children in the Florida demonstration were significantly less likely to fall, have contractures develop or worsen, have bed sores develop or worsen or develop a urinary tract infection than the control group (RWJF, 2006). The national PHB evaluation did not report any improvement in health status or clinical outcomes for PHB holders (Forder et al, 2012). However, fears that giving control to individuals would lead to a deterioration in their health status did not materialise.

The lack of improvement in clinical outcomes reported in the PHB evaluation is perhaps easily explained by the fact that improvements in health are not the central focus of a PHB for individuals. They value the approach for its ability to improve their overall quality of life and other priorities, such as their ability to work and carry out important family roles. These are often the outcomes that budget holders highlight in interviews and identify in care plans. This is reflected in the findings of the evaluation that reported a positive impact on care-related quality of life, psychological wellbeing and subjective wellbeing for PHB holders compared to the control group. Improvements in care-related quality of life justify the extension of PHBs because, as the evaluation states, 'people value care-related quality of life as measured using the ASCOT scale in that they are willing to exchange shorter life expectancy to avoid a longer life expectancy with poorer ASCOT-measured quality of life' (Forder et al, 2012, p 158).

Other studies also provide evidence to support the contribution of self-direction to wider quality of life outcomes. Participants in the Consumer Directed Care initiative in Australia reported improvements in several aspects of their quality of life after only a short period of time in the programme (Gordon et al, 2012). Self-directed programmes in mental health in the US have reported improvements in employment, education and training, housing stability and time spent in the community rather than in hospital or in the criminal justice system (Sullivan, 2006; Cook et al, 2008; Slade, 2012). While these are not controlled studies, the individual budget pilot, which did have a controlled design, also reported improvements in quality of life for participants with mental health needs compared to the control group, although this was counterbalanced by reports of poorer quality of life for older adults with an individual budget compared to the control group (Glendinning et al, 2008). Greater motivation, confidence and self-esteem have all been reported as outcomes of self-direction, and undeniably contribute to individual health and wellbeing (Health Foundation, 2010).

Cost-effectiveness

There are two levels at which we need to consider cost-effectiveness: the individual level and the system level. At the individual level, self-direction can improve value for money by creating better care outcomes for the same cost, as the PHB evaluation demonstrates. The evaluation concludes that overall PHBs are cost-effective on a care-related quality of life basis compared to conventional service delivery because individuals derive greater benefit for the same total cost of care (Forder et al, 2012).

There are also examples of PHBs reducing the costs of care by replacing expensive NHS services with less expensive alternatives. In the case of high value PHBs, the national evaluation finds that the total costs of care were lower for PHBs than for conventional service delivery (Forder et al, 2012). For example, analysis of high value CHC PHBs across five pilot sites found that, on average, PHBs cost 20 per cent less than the traditional care packages the same individuals had previously received (Alakeson and Duffy, 2011). One participant in the Northamptonshire PHB pilot for mental health spent £56,000 on NHS care in the year prior to having a PHB, including 67 inpatient days and nine contacts with the crisis team. In the first six months of having a PHB, she spent only £8,000 and had no inpatient stays.

These findings from the NHS echo similar findings from self-direction in social care. In the Florida Cash & Counseling program, parents of medically fragile children who were in control of their children's care spent 30 per cent less on nursing than those in the control group (Brown et al, 2007). The individual budget pilot reported a 6 per cent reduction in support costs and In Control's second phase programme reported a 9 per cent reduction in support costs compared to conventional service delivery. This fell from 12 per cent in In Control's first phase, but is more representative of the savings that can be expected from broad implementation (Glasby et al, 2010).

In several programmes internationally, cost neutrality or savings are built into the programme by reducing the value of the support available for self-direction compared to traditional service delivery. For example, in the Netherlands, PGBs are 25 per cent lower than the equivalent costs of traditional services on the grounds that overheads are lower (Alakeson, 2010). Where cost neutrality has not been built into the budget-setting methodology, programmes have run into trouble. For example, the Florida Self-directed Care program is run from within the Department of Children and Families' existing budget and, as such, is cost-neutral. However, an evaluation has revealed that more is spent per head on individuals in the Self-directed Care program than on those who are not. However, the extent to which individuals meet the outcomes they identify for themselves has not been routinely tracked, and it is not possible, therefore, to conclude whether or not the additional spending is, in fact, achieving greater value for money (OPPAGA, 2010).

The potential for cost-effectiveness at the individual level has been demonstrated: self-direction can reduce the costs of care for individuals or improve the benefit derived for the same cost. At the system level, for the NHS as a whole, the picture is less clear. Looking to social care for guidance, significant numbers have been able to access a personal budget without an increase in the overall costs of the system (Brindle, 2010). However, the impacts of personalisation for the NHS as a whole may be complex, as several studies internationally have revealed. If, as in the case of the Cash & Counseling demonstration in Arkansas, participants are better able to access the services to which they are eligible through self-direction than in the traditional system, self-direction will increase costs compared to traditional service delivery (Dale et al, 2004). The *Pfelgebudgets* demonstration in Germany found that, by providing greater access to paid care, personal budgets acted as a substitute for informal care without any discernible improvement in outcomes in the case of those who were receiving the existing cash payment for care. As such, any extension beyond the demonstration to existing cash recipient was likely to increase the costs of long-term care (Arntz and Thomsen, 2008b). In the Dutch PGB programme, costs grew because people who would not have taken up traditional services came into the government system when the option of a PGB was created (White, 2011). The PHB evaluation has shown that the costs of inpatient care are significantly lower for PHB holders compared to the control group but, unless this inpatient capacity is taken out of the NHS, the costs of the system as a whole will not fall.

From the perspective of those who choose to direct their own services, there is strong evidence that the approach is a cost-effective route to increase confidence and control, improve satisfaction with services and increase quality of life for those living with long-term conditions and disabilities. However, lessons from social care and international evidence remind us that positive outcomes from self-direction depend on how it is implemented (Health Foundation, 2010; Davidson et al, 2012). According to the PHB evaluation, pilot sites that offered flexibility and choice had a positive impact on wellbeing outcomes, while more restrictive approaches had a negative impact (Forder et al, 2012). Implementation is the subject of the next section, which sets out the steps in the PHB process and discusses the three types of infrastructure required for successful implementation of PHBs.

Section 2

Implementing personal health budgets

SIX

The personal health budget process

We saw in Section 1 that effective implementation has been critical in shaping positive outcomes for users of personal budgets in social care. Evidence from the PHB pilot reaches the same conclusion: implementation can make the difference between a positive and a negative experience for PHB holders and their families. The PHB evaluation highlights problems in some pilot sites with individuals not knowing how their budget was calculated or the value of their budget; some examples of inadequate support for planning; and a lack of transparency around the spending rules, leading to arbitrary approval or denial decisions and delays (Irvine at al, 2011; Davidson et al, 2012). Given its central importance, this section focuses on implementation and discusses the three types of infrastructure that are needed for PHBs in each of the following chapters: a system for allocating resources to individuals; a system of support for PHB holders which includes care planning; and the infrastructure for money management and monitoring. This chapter presents an overview of the PHB process. For anyone who has worked with personal budgets in social care, the process will feel familiar, but there are important differences given the clinical dimension to a PHB.

The seven-step personal health budget process

There are seven basic steps in the PHB process. These are common regardless of the condition for which a PHB is offered and are set out in Figure 6.1.

Step 1: Engaging individuals with PHBs. The first step is to engage potential PHB holders with the concept of a PHB, ensuring that they get good information and are able to make an informed decision about whether to take up the offer of a PHB. The decision to take up a PHB should always be voluntary, and it is absolutely critical that each person makes an active choice to have one as this is the start of the culture shift for the individual – from passive recipient of care to

Figure 6.1: An example of the personal health budget process for CHC

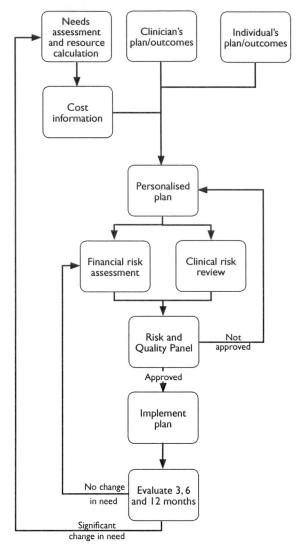

Source: This figure presents the steps in the process as set out by Central and Eastern Cheshire for CHC.

active participant. If the person is not engaged and informed at this stage, they will be a 'passenger' throughout the process and the PHB is less likely to succeed. Interviews with PHB holders three months after joining the programme found people still struggling with the concept of personalisation as they were used to professionals telling them what was best (Irvine et al, 2011).

The point at which individuals are offered a PHB is critical. As part of the pilot programme, a small group of individuals who had suffered a stroke were offered a PHB while they were still seriously ill and, consequently, found the process stressful (Davidson et al, 2012, p 55). Similarly, individuals with mental health or substance misuse issues may come into contact with services at a point of crisis when the priority is to stabilise their condition. They need to get beyond this point to be able to think about their ongoing treatment and support needs and how a PHB could help. Leaving open the possibility of a PHB so that individuals can take up one when they are ready rather than only making them available at a fixed point in the care pathway is central to making them inclusive and effective.

Step 2: Identifying the value of a PHB. Once an individual has opted for a PHB, it is necessary to identify the cash value of the PHB to which that person is entitled once everyone has a clear understanding of the person's needs. PHBs tend to focus on a particular set of needs or a particular aspect of care where choice and creativity could make a real difference. For example, an individual with substance misuse problems may receive a PHB for substance misuse treatment and recovery but continue to see their GP and receive NHS services for any physical health conditions that they may also have. An individual with motor neurone disease will continue to see their neurologist and GP but may be offered a PHB to maintain mobility and support their ongoing independence instead of receiving traditional physiotherapy or occupational therapy.

There are different ways in which the cash value of a PHB can be set which will be discussed in the next chapter, but it is important that this process recognises an individual's needs, the needs of any carers and the strengths and assets the individual has to contribute. Resources should not be allocated purely according to clinical need. Individuals should be made aware of the value of their PHB before any planning takes place.

Step 3: Care planning. The PHB allocation provides the starting point for an individual to develop a care plan that identifies the goals that individual has for their health and wellbeing and how those goals can be met. The care plan can be developed with informal support from friends and family or with the support of an independent broker. Clinicians need to work closely with individuals from the earliest part of the planning process to ensure that clinical needs are met in ways that fit with an individual's wider goals and family situation. Care planning is discussed in detail in Chapter 8.

Step 4: Approving the care plan. The care plan is signed off from a financial and clinical point of view. Broadly, plans are approved on the basis that the services and supports chosen will help meet the outcomes set out in the plan, do not exceed the value of the PHB and do not put the individual or those working with them at an unacceptable level of risk.

Step 5: Choosing how the money is held. Individuals can exercise as much or as little direct control over the money in their PHB as they choose. If their CCG has direct payment powers, they can receive their PHB as a direct payment that they manage with support. They can use a third party to hold the money and employ people on their behalf, or the money can be held as a notional budget by commissioners. The options for how the money is held is discussed further in Chapter 9. Whichever way they choose to receive the money, individuals should be able to exercise control over the decisions that matter most to them.

Step 6: Putting the plan into action. With decisions about the money made, the services and supports in the care plan can be put into action and the individual can get on with living life. Irrespective of how the money is held, individuals and families should have as much choice and control as they wish over how their services and supports are put in place, including making decisions about rates of pay, staff competencies and back-up plans.

Step 7: The review process. The care plan should be formally reviewed at least annually or in line with the standard review process for the condition in question. When a PHB is first put in place, an early initial review can be helpful to check things are progressing well. The focus of the review should be to judge whether the outcomes identified in the care plan are being met. If an individual's needs change significantly, they will need to take part in a reassessment that may lead to a change in the value of their PHB.

While the steps in the PHB process have been set out in a linear fashion for the sake of clarity, it is important to remember that, in reality, the process is ongoing. As individuals gain experience with their PHB, they will have new ideas about how best to meet their needs and make different choices. The process needs to be able to accommodate this, for example, by providing individuals with enough flexibility to make changes in their care plan between formal reviews. Some individuals may prefer to take on control incrementally over time as their confidence with PHBs grows. For example, they may opt for a PHB but continue to use a care agency to deliver their care at the outset, and step by step, switch to hiring their own staff. One of the conclusions from the national evaluation is that 'information giving and decision-making about PHBs need to be conceived as an ongoing process not a one-off event' (Irvine et al, 2011, p 26).

Agreeing a local framework for personal health budgets

The seven steps described earlier provide a basic overview of the PHB process that can be applied anywhere. In reality, however, they need to be set within a transparent, well-understood framework that is agreed locally. Doing so will avoid issues cropping up later in the day that can undermine the benefits of PHBs. Creating a local framework needs to involve everyone who has a stake in the process from the outset, including commissioners, clinicians, individuals and their families, finance officers and local authority colleagues. As with any major change in the way in which a large, healthcare system operates, securing board level support for the implementation of PHBs is a critical part of developing a local framework. It will be difficult for mid-level managers and frontline staff to overcome resistance to new ways of working without being able to call on senior level support.

The purpose of a local implementation framework is to clarify how the concept of a PHB that has been developed nationally and refined through the pilot programme is implemented in a particular local area. Developing a local implementation framework provides an opportunity to reach agreement early on about the guidelines governing PHBs. In the absence of a clear local framework, several pilot sites found that when they consulted stakeholders about PHBs a year into implementation, there were many differences of opinion about their purpose and the policies governing their use. These differences of opinion acted as a barrier to effective implementation (Brewis et al, 2012).

As discussed in Chapter 1, there are only a few national guidelines governing how PHBs can be used and, therefore, the majority need to be determined locally. Once set, guidelines need to be communicated clearly to all interested parties and information about them made available to ensure transparency. Establishing rules at the outset does not, however, mean that they are fixed. They will need to change as PHBs evolve locally. The box below identifies the four critical areas where guidelines should be established early on.

Setting the 'rules' for personal health budgets
Establish guidelines for the following early on and allow them to evolve as the PHB programme develops:

1. How PHBs will be calculated for specific conditions and how much will be available based on what criteria.
2. The 'rules' for how flexibly the money in a PHB can be used. This avoids the need for decisions to be taken on a case-by-case basis that can be subjective and time-consuming.
3. The criteria against which care plans will be signed off and who is responsible for the clinical and financial sign-off.
4. How spending will be monitored and the frequency with which care plans will be reviewed and their effectiveness evaluated.

Source: Brewis et al (2012)

As the national evaluation highlights, the failure to agree local guidelines can result in care plans being turned down without clear justification, causing frustration and disappointment (Forder et al, 2012, p 164) – iPads and other gadgets have been a case in point. Individuals receiving CHC who are paralysed and largely confined to the house have included iPads and similar gadgets within their care plans as a means of remaining remotely in contact with friends and family. Stephen's story (see page vi) highlights some of the benefits that technology can bring in such cases. In some pilot sites, these care plans have been turned down by commissioners, even when a clear justification has been given for how an iPad can meet an individual's needs and when no prior rule has prohibited their purchase. This has been largely because commissioners have felt uncomfortable signing off public money for something that could be deemed a 'luxury'. However, for individuals, the seemingly arbitrary nature of the decision has created disappointment, having submitted a plan in good faith. In some cases, a lack of clarity over local guidelines can cause lengthy waits that undermine people's satisfaction with PHBs.

This chapter has outlined the basic steps in the PHB process and highlighted the importance of setting this process within a clear local framework. The remaining three chapters in this section focus on the three types of infrastructure needed to deliver PHBs at a local level: a system for allocating resources; a system for supporting budget holders during care planning and throughout the entire PHB process; and options for holding and managing the money in a PHB. On average, pilot sites invested around £146,000 over two years in developing this infrastructure (Jones et al, 2011, p 2). While these costs have to be found from existing budgets, effective implementation pays its way in the long run through quicker, more efficient processes, greater satisfaction and, ultimately, better outcomes.

SEVEN

How to set a personal health budget

One of the five essential features of a PHB is that individuals should know upfront how much they have to spend in advance of starting to plan how best to meet their needs (DH, 2012e). This transparency makes care planning more effective, as discussed in the next chapter. Therefore, in order to implement PHBs, it is necessary to develop a process for allocating NHS resources to each eligible individual in a way that is fair between individuals and that ensures each person can meet their needs from within their allocated resources. It is important to remember that the allocation of resources to an individual is not the process that determines eligibility for a PHB. It simply determines the level of the PHB once an individual has been assessed as eligible. For example, in the context of NHS CHC, the decision support tool (DST) is the national eligibility framework. If individuals are eligible for CHC on the basis of their score on the DST, a separate allocation system subsequently determines the value of their PHB.

Findings from the national evaluation highlight a significant lack of clarity among participants about the level of their PHB and how it was determined. Three months after having signed up for a PHB, few participants knew how much was in their budget (Irvine et al, 2011), and even nine months into the pilot, a minority did not understand that a PHB was their own personalised allocation of funding. They did not know how much was in their budget, how much they had already spent, or even whether they had a budget in place (Davidson et al, 2012).

The evaluation results emphasise the need to get this stage of the PHB process right. Experience from personal budgets in social care cautions against making the allocation system too complicated. The first system that was developed in 2003 was one A4 page long. There are now local authorities with resource allocation systems that are 40 pages long, complex, restrictive of choice and costly (Duffy, 2011a). Keeping it simple is essential to the success of PHBs. After all, the initial budget amount around which an individual plans is only an indicative amount; it is a guide for care planning. It can be approximate in its accuracy rather than exact. A final budget amount is agreed at the point of final sign-off alongside the care plan.

Approaches to allocating resources to personal health budgets

The PHB pilot sites generally adopted one of three approaches to resource allocation: one-off payments; allocating resources on the basis of existing services; or needs-based budgets.

One-off payments

One-off payments have been used successfully in several pilot sites to provide additional impetus to the management of a long-term condition. For example, in the Norfolk PHB pilot, individuals with dementia were given an additional £500 on a one-off basis with which to buy services and supports that would help them manage their condition and that were not available from the NHS, for example, a garden kneeler to help an older person continue gardening. One-off payments have also been piloted in adult mental health services and have been found to act as a spur to recovery (Coyle, 2009).

One-off payments can be an easy way for commissioners and providers to experiment with choice and control for individuals. However, lower value PHBs have been found to have a less positive impact on care-related quality of life and psychological wellbeing than PHBs of more than £1,000 (Forder et al, 2012, p 10). Furthermore, they are generally offered on top of existing services. This makes them hard to sustain in the tight financial climate currently faced by the NHS, and they do not sufficiently demonstrate that individual choice and control can improve outcomes over traditional service delivery. Rather, if individuals improve, it is on the basis of receiving extra support. Therefore, one-off payments should be treated as a place to start rather than the best approach to allocating resources for PHBs.

Allocating resources on the basis of existing services

Several pilot sites allocated resources based on the traditional service package that an individual would otherwise have received, or based on the services the individual had used in the previous year. This was also a common approach in social care in the early days of personal budgets. Starting from the value of existing services can be an easier way to get going than developing a system from scratch that allocates resources on the basis of need. The downside to this approach is that existing biases are built into the PHB system. For example, if the current system over-supports individuals, this will be built into the allocation system for PHBs. Equally, if the current system does not emphasise prevention in its use of resources, it can be more difficult to create this shift in health behaviour with a budget based on existing patterns of service use.

However, where a PHB is offered in place of a single NHS service, such as physiotherapy or psychological therapy, cashing out the value of the existing service is an effective way of establishing a PHB. For example, in Eastern and Coastal Kent, individuals could opt for a PHB instead of 12 sessions of cognitive behavioural therapy provided by the local NHS trust as Yve did (see Yve's story). Commissioners worked closely with the trust to identify the cost per person of the improving access to psychological therapy (IAPT) step three service. The identified cost per individual of the 12 sessions offered through the IAPT service was used as the cash value of a PHB for those who opted to control their own care (Walton, 2012).

Yve's story

Yve is a mother of two who has spent most of her career working in NHS administration and is the proud owner of a dog, Bailey, who has a penchant for eating handbags. For many years, Yve lived with depression and was unaware that her life could be different. When she felt low, she struggled to leave the house, did not want to see friends and lost interest in life in general.

Fortunately, through her job in the NHS, Yve was able to get eight sessions of counselling a year to help with her depression, but she was never able to go back to the same counsellor, and once the eight sessions were over, she had to wait another year to get more help. Her GP had prescribed anti-depressants and had encouraged her to get a dog. Bailey gave her a reason to get up in the morning which helped her depression. But when her last eight weeks of counselling ran out and she felt she hadn't made enough improvement, she returned to her GP in search of a new solution. Ideally, she wanted to be well enough to stop taking the anti-depressants. They didn't help her deal with her problems. They just deadened everything.

Her GP referred her to the psychological therapy service at her local NHS hospital but there was six to 18 month waiting list for individual therapy. She was offered a PHB as an alternative and, with the support of a health broker, put together a care plan. With her PHB, Yve was able to go back to a counsellor she had worked with in the past whose approach had benefited her. Since she already had a relationship with the counsellor, she was able to negotiate a discount so she could have more sessions for the same money. She was also interested in using reflexology to relax and deal with stress and was able to negotiate a good deal with a practitioner. Yve was also becoming more isolated and wanted to do something that would help her socialise. In the past she had started to learn hands-on healing and decided to try this as a route to meeting new people. Her reflexologist taught Reiki groups, which allowed her to mix with others as well as learning a new skill that could help with her depression.

Yve feels lucky to have had the opportunity to use a PHB and feels that her life has changed dramatically as a result. She has rebuilt her relationship with her mother that lay at the root of many of her problems. She has a new sense of self-worth, has made new friends and is going out and enjoying life again. She has gone back to work covering maternity leave but is hopeful that this may turn into a permanent job. She has stopped taking anti-depressants and is more positive about things. "I feel like I was one of the lucky ones. I am so grateful", she said about her PHB experience.

Source: Author's interview with Yve Beautridge, June 2012

Needs-based resource allocation

The most common approach to determining the value of a PHB is to allocate resources on the basis of need. This chapter gives two examples from the pilot programme of how sites have allocated resources for two different services. These are just examples, however; there is no standard approach for how this should be done, and most pilot sites updated their approach many times during the pilot programme as they learned more about how people use their budgets. Ideally, a PHB should include resources to support an individual's wider wellbeing needs and not simply the minimum budgetary amount to ensure their clinical needs are met. In the example from Croydon, the resource allocation system includes rebuilding relationships with friends and family and community integration, both of which are likely to support an individual's ongoing recovery from substance misuse but that go beyond a strict interpretation of clinical need. Whichever approach is taken, it is important to keep it as simple as possible and to provide a transparent account of how the value of a PHB is calculated.

Croydon's resource allocation system for substance misuse treatment and recovery

Croydon has developed a resource allocation system that allocates funding against the following domains through a supported self-assessment questionnaire that individuals complete with a care navigator:

- Opiate use stabilisation (£3,010 max)
- Ongoing prescribing of opiate substitute (£2,590 max)
- Detoxification (£7,000 max)
- Help with symptoms of withdrawal (£210 max)
- Practical barriers/obstacles to treatment (£490 max)
- Risk and harm reduction (£700 max)
- Helping individuals to change their behaviour/use of substances (£490 max)
- Emotional and mental health (£490 max)
- Repairing damage to key relationships with family and friends (£700 max)
- Community integration and community life (£700 max)

Responses to statements/descriptors under each of these domains produce a score that is then linked to an allocation of resources. Not all individuals will attract resources in all of the above domains. An individual's PHB is the sum total of the allocations in each domain and the maximum indicative budget an individual can get is £16,380. The domains do not restrict how a PHB is used. The care planning process helps the budget holder to make best use of the PHB alongside universal services and other community resources to pursue recovery (Colhoun and Porter, 2012).

NHS Oxfordshire's budget setting tool for continuing healthcare

Much like Croydon, the budget setting approach used by NHS Oxfordshire does not focus solely on clinical needs but includes wider aspects of health and wellbeing. As a first step, information about an individual's clinical needs are identified using the DST as part of the CHC eligibility process and are recorded in a service requisition. This clearly states the type and frequency of care and support required to meet the individual's healthcare needs. On the basis of these needs, the budget tool calculates the cost of the support required by the individual using locally set rates for care agencies or directly hired personal assistants.

In addition to the costs of support required to meet an individual's healthcare needs, the tool adds any other care and support costs that an individual might need to live life, not just meet basic health needs, such as the costs of leisure and educational activities. These are recorded under 'Other charges' in the tool shown (see Table 7.1).

If an indicative budget is calculated on the basis of the number of hours of hands–on support required, as is often the case in CHC, the budget needs to include additional employer, insurance and training costs such as sick pay, the cost of criminal background checks if required, recruitment costs and public liability insurance. In addition, where care packages are large and require a significant amount of management from a family member, as is often the case with CHC, the Department of Health is proposing that a fee can be paid to family

Table 7.1: NHS Oxfordshire's resource allocation system for CHC

Care package requirements (from service requisition)	Unit measure	Unit cost (£)	Units per week	Cost per week (£)
Care agencies (average rates)				
Weekday daytime rate	per hour	17.80	0.00	0.00
Weekend daytime rate	per hour	20.70	0.00	0.00
Waking nights weekdays (9-hour night)	per hour	17.18	0.00	0.00
Waking nights weekends (9-hour night)	per hour	20.29	0.00	0.00
Sleeping nights	per night	70.00	0.00	0.00
Live-in carer	per week	800.00	0.00	0.00
Employed staff				
Live-in care	per week	500.00		0.00
Weekday daytime rate	per hour	8.50	0.00	0.00
Weekend daytime rate	per hour	11.05	0.00	0.00
Waking night (9 hours)	per hour	10.00		0.00
Sleeping night (9 hours)	per night	50.00	0.00	0.00
Other charges				
Transport				0.00
Supplies	per week	7.00		0.00
Day centre (meals not included)	per day			0.00
Employee on-costs (live-in)	per week	133.00	0.00	0.00
Employee on-costs (daytime)	per hour	2.26	0.00	0.00
Employee on-costs (weekend)	per hour	2.94	0.00	0.00
Employee on-costs (waking night)	per hour	2.66	0.00	0.00
Employee on-costs (sleeping nights)	per night	13.30	0.00	0.00
Total cost per week				£0.00

Table 7.1: continued

	Unit measure (per day, per shift etc, per hour etc)	Unit cost (£)	Per year	Cost per year (£)
Annual charges/start-up costs				
Employers/public liability	per year	99.00	0	0.00
PA clinical indemnity insurance	per year			0.00
Bank holiday supplements	per day	0.00	0	0.00
Training	per day	66.00	0	0.00
	per half-day	36.00	0	0.00
	per half-day	36.00		0.00
PA rate for training (+ on-costs)	per hour	10.76	0	0.00
Recruitment	per year	500.00		
Annual charges				0.00
Annual budget	52 weeks			0.00
Average weekly cost (for authorisation purposes only)				0.00
Respite allocation	**Unit measure**	**Unit cost (£)**	**Per year**	**Cost per year (£)**
	per week	0.00	0	0.00

members to cover their management time (DH, 2013). Therefore, as a final step, the Oxfordshire budget tool adds in employee on-costs, set-up costs, training costs and any respite costs related to family carers (Cattermole, 2012a).

Resource allocation and Payment by Results

Payment by Results (PbR) is the activity-based payment system in the NHS that allows commissioners to pay providers a national price (or tariff) for around 1,400 different activities (or currencies). PbR was first introduced in 2003 to promote efficiency and support patient choice. It is increasingly being used to promote best practice models of care by fixing tariffs according to the costs of best practice approaches. PbR currently covers the majority of acute healthcare in hospitals and some outpatient procedures. Around 30 per cent of the funding allocated to local commissioners is spent via PbR and national tariffs account for around 60 per cent of a hospital trust's income (DH, 2011a).

As part of expanding PbR to other areas, pathway rather than activity-based currencies are currently being developed. These set a tariff for a year of care for people with long-term conditions at different levels of need. Pathway currencies have already been introduced for cystic fibrosis and paediatric diabetes. Other work is being done to extend PbR to mental health, and community services are under consideration. Pathway currencies potentially provide an established approach to resource allocation for PHBs.

In mental health, PbR is based on 21 care clusters. For example, clusters 1-4 include all non-psychotic mild, moderate and severe mental health conditions and clusters 11-13 include severe, ongoing mental health conditions with psychosis. Commissioners will purchase services on the basis of the number of people they have locally within each cluster, with each person attracting a locally determined price per cluster (DH, 2012f). While there are clear tensions between the diagnosis-based, clinical approach to care clusters and the broader sense of health and wellbeing underpinning PHBs, in Northamptonshire, mental health PbR is being used as the basis for allocating resources for PHBs. Following a cluster assessment or review, each individual receiving mental health services is assigned to a care cluster. If individuals opt to control their own services instead of receiving a traditional care package, the cluster cost becomes their indicative budget and the starting point for care planning (Cattermole, 2012b).

Mainstreaming PHBs in this way by embedding them in the infrastructure being developed for PbR rather than developing a separate approach to resource allocation may make it more likely that PHBs will flourish in the NHS. As PbR and PHBs develop, the fit between the two systems will have to be closely monitored. Given that PbR only allocates resources on the basis of a clinical assessment and does not focus on wider health and wellbeing, there is a risk that the resources allocated through this approach are insufficient for individuals to achieve broader outcomes, while actively managing their health. Furthermore, there is a risk that PbR will reduce the flexibility of PHBs if the care pathways underpinning PbR are used to limit individual choice.

Developing an approach to allocating resources for PHBs can be technically challenging, and keeping it simple can be tricky. However, it is important not to place undue emphasis on the budget. It is an important step in the process for individuals to know how much they have to plan with, but it is the care planning phase of the process that is the centrepiece of a PHB. The budget alone is not sufficient. It is just the starting point for a different kind of conversation between individuals and clinicians about how to better manage an individual's health and wellbeing in order to live a more fulfilling life. As we will see in the next chapter, care planning is at the heart of changing the balance of power in the NHS between the learned expertise of professionals and the lived experience of individuals and families.

EIGHT

Getting the most out of care planning

Care planning is intended to form a central part of the management of long-term conditions in the NHS, and the majority of people with a long-term condition report having a care planning discussion with their health professional (Singh and Ham, 2006). However, it is still the case that care planning is largely professionally driven. Professionals often start mentally slotting individuals into available services based on the written results of an assessment before even meeting or talking to the individual in question. Professionals only have so many service options to work with, and individuals have to fit into one. The flexibility of a PHB means that individuals do not have to slot in where they do not quite fit. It is possible to really individualise the care planning process to include tailor-made goals and choices.

The care planning process for PHBs is driven by the individual, and the plan can take whatever form the individual chooses and is written in the individual's own words. That said, individuals who are in receipt of a PHB can have significant health problems that need to be well managed as an integral part of them enjoying a good life. Access to clinical knowledge and advice remains important. However, individual choices and preferences need to be factored into the way in which clinical care is delivered and who delivers it.

The common failure to take medication as prescribed often stems from the negative effects of prescribed medicine on facets of life that individuals consider important, such as their role as a parent or employee. These activities have been described as 'personal medicine' – the everyday activities that can be a source of motivation and have significant therapeutic value. A conflict between professionally recommended treatment and 'personal medicine' arises when medical professionals fail to consider the preferences and life circumstances of individuals when planning care (Deegan, 2005). In working with individuals and families, clinicians need to acknowledge and respect their expertise and work with them to make a reality of their choices rather than dismissing alternatives as too risky and not clinically proven. In an ideal process, a clinician should have been involved enough in the development of a care plan not to be surprised by what is in it when it is submitted for approval. Unusual choices should already have been discussed and their motivation and value understood well before the point of approval (Alakeson, 2012). The benefits and challenges for clinicians of working with PHBs are discussed further in Section 3.

The domains of a care plan for personal health budgets

The overriding purpose of a care plan is to determine whether the goals an individual has for their health and well being are likely to be met by the things listed in their plan, whether any potential risks have been identified and are adequately managed with back-up plans in place and whether the plan comes in under the indicative budget amount. There is no standard form for a care plan, but each plan should capture the following information to facilitate sign-off:

- Details of the individual's health condition and any care and treatment currently being received. In some cases, this information will be contained in a prior assessment. It is important that it is fed into the care plan to ensure that an individual's health needs are adequately met. In some pilot sites, a summary of the clinical assessment was provided to support effective care planning.
- The impact of the individual's health condition on them physically, emotionally and socially. This situates the individual and their clinical needs within a broader life context and highlights how the condition affects other aspects of their lives.
- What is working and not working in the individual's life. This identifies aspects of the individual's life and care that they would like to maintain and those aspects that they would like to improve. For example, an individual's pain may be well managed but they might feel isolated at home and want to increase their social activity.
- What is important to the individual. This may be captured in the previous section, but it is critical that the plan clearly records the things that are important to the individual so that the goals and purchases that follow can be fully understood by anyone signing off the plan.
- The outcomes the individual wants to meet and how they intend to meet them. This can include universal services, free community resources and informal support as well as paid for goods and services.
- Possible risks need to be recorded and plans identified for how they will be managed. If an individual employs their own staff, back-up plans for staff illness and holidays need to be included.
- Details of how the individual wants to hold the money. This is discussed in detail in Chapter 9.
- An action plan for how the different parts of the plan will be put in place, including who is responsible for putting in place each element of the plan.

Source: Brewis et al (2012)

The care planning process

As with many aspects of a PHB, care planning is not a linear process and budget holders may develop several versions of their plan before they are satisfied. This can often taken longer and be a more time-consuming process than professionally-led care planning, but it pays for itself many times over in the medium term, with care packages being less likely to break down and individuals being more likely to stick to care plans because they have taken the lead in developing them (Reynolds, 2012). The following are the basic steps in the process to get from an indicative budget to an approved final budget and plan:

1. Once an individual has an indicative budget, they can start to develop their care plan. At this point, individuals need to be informed about the local guidelines discussed in Chapter 6 to help them understand what is expected of them and what they can expect from the process.
2. At the beginning of the care planning process, individuals should be offered support to complete their plan if they want it. Most pilot sites found that independent support was more effective than case managers or other clinicians trying to support individuals, as Dr Greg Rogers, a GP from Kent, discusses on page **98**. Information, advice and support are discussed in more detail later. Some individuals will be able to complete their plan on their own or with help from friends and family, and will not need professional support.
3. As discussed earlier, it is important that clinicians are involved in discussions from early on in the process. A good approach can be for a clinician and an independent support broker or project manager to jointly visit a potential budget holder to discuss the outcomes they might want to pursue with their PHB.
4. The completed plan is submitted for approval and sign-off. Plans will usually be signed off by a health professional from a clinical perspective and by a commissioner from a financial perspective. The clearer the guidelines are upfront as to what purchases are allowed and the basis on which plans will be approved, the simpler the sign-off procedure can be. This is discussed further later.
5. Once the plan is approved, a final budget amount is agreed. An appeals process needs to be put in place to deal with individuals who feel that their case has not been handled fairly. Once again, clear upfront rules will reduce the likelihood of appeals (Brewis et al, 2012).

Planning for fluctuating conditions

Some long-term conditions have unpredictable fluctuations that can be difficult to manage. Other people with fluctuating conditions will know at what points their condition is likely to deteriorate and what the triggers are. In the same way as budget holders need to plan for other risks, some can plan for these periods of fluctuation by setting aside money from their budget. In their care plan, they can record the care and support they require when their condition deteriorates, who can help them put the necessary support in place and what the signs are that indicate that they are getting worse. For example, someone with arthritis may be able to manage day-to-day life relatively well, but when their condition flares up, they may struggle to get out of bed. They could set aside some money from their PHB to pay for additional childcare or a personal assistant during these periods when they struggle to cope.

Advanced planning can also facilitate choice in periods when individuals lack the capacity to make independent decisions. Under the 2005 Mental Capacity Act a person lacks capacity if they are unable to make a decision because of an impairment or a disturbance in the functioning of the mind or brain. Adults with mental health conditions, for example, may experience crisis periods when they are not best placed to plan their care. However, planning in advance when they are well and setting aside part of their PHB to deal with crises can reduce the need for hospitalisation and significantly improve their overall experience of care (Alakeson and Perkins, 2012). For example, some people find a short stay in a bed and breakfast or increased support at home a particularly effective form of respite when their mental health worsens. This has been tried with great success by the mental health charity, Mind, in Norwich using social care personal budgets. Individuals have been supported to remain at home during a period of crisis when they may otherwise have gone into hospital by providing them with visits two or three times a day and a worker to stay overnight if necessary. For risk management purposes, a back-up plan is developed with the individual, and a crisis team remains on standby (Alakeson et al, 2013).

Older adults with dementia or at the end of life may similarly lack the capacity to plan how to use a PHB at the time they become eligible. The opportunity to develop a care plan in advance that can be put into action when they become eligible for support can maximise the benefits of a PHB and provide reassurance that the way in which the

PHB is being used reflects the individual's choices rather than simply those of a carer (Exley et al, 2011).

For conditions that fluctuate but nevertheless require significant levels of care and support on a day-to-day basis, which is the case for many people in receipt of CHC, it may not be possible to manage fluctuations effectively unless additional resources can be made available. Resources from an existing PHB cannot be targeted at periods of fluctuation unless an individual goes without necessary care and support at other times to build up a 'rainy day' fund. Given that PHBs have been shown to reduce the costs of inpatient care compared to traditional NHS services, a proportion of these costs could be added to a PHB to help such individuals manage fluctuations that may otherwise result in more costly interventions.

Although long-term conditions are progressive, some individuals may enjoy periods of improvement, and the amount of support they can receive may reduce accordingly. This is not particular to PHBs but is made more transparent when individuals are allocated a sum of money, not a service. There is concern that PHBs could encourage dependency because individuals seek to hold on to the money they have and the goods and services they have been able to buy with it. Two things are important to address any risk of dependency. First, it is important that individuals understand from the outset that their PHB is not an ongoing entitlement, and that as they progress, their support will reduce. Most people want to see their health improve and their lives get back on track and, therefore, there should be little resistance to this. Second, it is essential to help people rebuild social support as part of their care plan to enable them to move on without fear as their health starts to improve, as we saw in Chapter 1, in the case of Alex.

Information, advice and support

Putting in place information, advice and support for budget holders is a critical part of the infrastructure for PHBs and is central to ensuring that the approach works for all budget holders and not just those who are most able. As we saw in Chapter 2, the availability of information, advice and support for personal budget holders in social care has been highly variable across local authorities, and has had a significant impact on the ability of individuals to make best use of their personal budget. The PHB evaluation found that most people were satisfied with the information and support that they were offered, although those who were more reluctant to ask questions were more likely to want more information to be freely available. The area where information was felt to be most valuable was in providing examples and stories of how other people had used their budget as a source of inspiration, particularly others with the same condition. However, the final evaluation report cautions against a prescriptive approach:

> ... it was important that such lists [of suggestions] were treated as suggestions only, rather than constituting a definitive menu, otherwise participants felt uncomfortable about or inhibited from requesting items they thought would benefit them but were not on the list. (Forder et al, 2012, p 163)

Examples and stories that give new budget holders a sense of the possible can be particularly valuable for those who have been receiving services for a long time for whom it may be more challenging to think about how their care could look different.

As well as access to information, it is important that individuals have access to support throughout the care planning process. There is a tendency to focus on the support needed to write a care plan, but PHB holders have emphasised the value of support throughout the process from somebody who knows them well (Brewis and Fitzgerald, 2012). In writing a care plan individuals often need to reveal intimate details about themselves, things that they may not have shared with many other people. It is important, therefore, that they have time to develop a rapport and a good degree of trust with whomever is supporting them. Several pilot sites experimented with having clinicians support individuals to write a plan, but this was not very successful. Clinicians felt that the process was too time-consuming and they often struggled to break out of traditional services and be creative with care planning. There are three broad options for how to provide support:

* Independent support brokers have been used extensively. A support broker is an independent guide whose purpose is to ensure that individuals can live the life they choose. Brokers respond to an individual's priorities, not the priorities of the NHS. They are often employed by the third sector and tend not to be health professionals, but are skilled in working with individuals and knowing how to find out about different options outside of statutory services, including free options in the community. Many local authorities use independent support brokers to work with personal budget holders, and it is advisable to tap into existing resources such as this to minimise implementation costs (Dowson, 2007).

- Paid peer support can be an effective alternative to support brokerage, particularly in areas such as mental health and substance misuse where the stigma that comes with the condition is still highly corrosive of people's hope and sense of possibility. The mentorship of a peer can make all the difference to helping someone move beyond their illness to re-engage with life and their community. Texas Self-directed Care, for example, uses paid peers as recovery coaches to support participants through the programme, including the planning phase.
- Informal support can also be a valuable resource. This can be from friends and family and also from other PHB holders who volunteer on a reciprocal basis to plan with someone else. One approach to developing a local network of informal support for planning would be to ask all PHB holders when they complete their plan if they would be prepared to support someone else to plan.

These three options create a tiered offer of support that can meet different levels of need. Making PHBs sustainable will depend on providing appropriate levels of support rather than over-supporting people. Support should be provided on the assumption that individuals will move down the levels of support over time as they themselves become more skilled and will not always require a professional broker. Furthermore, it is important to recognise that some people will be able to plan on their own from the outset. This is borne out by the evaluation that shows that those who already knew what they wanted to do with their PHB were able to plan independently (Irvine et al, 2011). Providing support to those who do not need it will only make the system more expensive and potentially deskill individuals who can manage on their own (Duffy and Fulton, 2009).

Signing off plans

The process for signing off care plans should remain proportionate to the clinical risks and costs involved in the plan. For the process to work smoothly, the most important factor is to establish a clear set of guidelines that remove as much of the subjectivity around approval as possible. If a plan does not include any prohibited items, clearly demonstrates how the purchases meet the goals identified by the individual, adequately addresses health needs and is within budget, the plan should be approved. Subjective decision making is more time-consuming. It allows individual moral judgements into the decision-making process and can lead to significant disappointment for budget holders who are unclear why their plan has not been approved.

The simplest approach to sign-off is to keep approval as close to the front line as possible. This reduces bureaucracy and ensures that the person responsible for signing off the plan knows the individual well and can easily understand the rationale for different purchases. In one pilot site, for example, the CHC clinical lead signed off all the plans from a clinical perspective and took them to the lead commissioner for financial sign-off. However, in some areas individuals have been reluctant to take sole responsibility for sign-off. In this case, it can be helpful to establish a small review group of up to three people. Individuals can present their own plans which makes it more likely that reviewers will gain a full understanding of how the purchases listed in the plan relate to individual goals and a person's broader family and social context.

Larger panels similar to the panels traditionally used for exceptional expenditure in the NHS have the tendency to become bureaucratic and costly, driven by the views of the most sceptical panel member. All too often the costs of the time of the five senior people sitting on the panel far outweigh the cost of the item the panel is debating (Cattermole, 2012c, p 8). A proportion of PHB holders in the evaluation reported that the approval process was lengthy and complex, and there were significant delays leading to disappointment (Davidson et al, 2012, p 31).

A GP's view of personal health budgets

'Doctors are the very worst for having this patient-led. It's not their fault.... Doctors have got too much knowledge and power and it's all clinical. Brokers were like neutral outsiders, more like paid counsellors really, coming in, leading and guiding. And it was so different, quite visibly different.'

Greg Rogers is a GP in Kent. He became involved with the PHB pilot in Eastern and Coastal Kent for CHC, mental health and maternity care as a result of a personalised care planning pilot that he was involved in at the time through the strategic health authority.

With clinical staff responsible for developing personalised care plans, Greg found that it was difficult to achieve high quality plans. Care plans were all too often disease management plans rather than plans focused on what the patient wanted to achieve. According to Greg, GPs are not trained in motivational interviewing. They have too much knowledge and power and patients are too ready to defer to doctors because they believe doctors know everything. As a result, the conversation moves away too easily from how a patient wants to improve their life to medical complaints and clinical care. Simple desires such as wanting to go to the shops once a week or to go swimming that could significantly improve an individual's quality of life are rarely addressed.

As a result of his experience with the personalised care planning pilot, Greg teamed up with the PHB pilot and saw what a difference the health broker involved in the pilot could make to the planning process. Unencumbered by clinical training, the broker was better placed to develop a truly personal care plan. In Greg's view the core of a PHB is the quality of the care plan. Genuine person-centred care planning is outside of the comfort zone of most GPs and outside their skills and training. While GPs need to remain involved and should be involved in sign-off, Greg's view is that third sector organisations are better placed to lead care planning. Well-trained, accredited brokers overseen by clinical providers can do a much better job than doctors or other clinical staff. This could also be a way to sustain many third sector and community organisations that are currently struggling as a result of public sector cuts.

Through his contact with the pilot, Greg learned how positively people felt about having a PHB. They rarely chose to do anything dangerous with their money. Going to the gym instead of physiotherapy is not risky and makes sense. On the contrary, PHBs for CHC and depression, for example, could have a massive impact and save the NHS money. While some GPs will be concerned about raising expectations that can't be met, in Greg's view, the pilot has shown that many of the things that people want can be achieved if the question is asked. For example, it turned out that a woman who was receiving renal dialysis wanted to swim once a week but her GP was unlikely to ever ask her the right question to find that out.

In Greg's opinion, many GPs would support PHBs because most recognise that long-term conditions are untreatable and progressive and they would generally be in favour of something that was cost-neutral and could improve people's quality of life and wellbeing. The major challenge that Greg sees in implementing PHBs is the current financial climate in the NHS. It would be much easier to implement a new initiative if there was more money available to invest in change and provide well-staffed teams to lead implementation.

Source: Author's interview with Dr Greg Rogers, November 2012

We have now discussed two elements of the infrastructure required to successfully implement PHBs: the process for allocating resources and the support needed for PHB holders, including information, advice and support for care planning. The next chapter looks at the infrastructure required for individuals to manage their PHB and for commissioners to monitor how effectively it is used.

NINE

Managing and monitoring the money

Changes in legislation introduced as part of the PHB pilot made it legally possible for the first time for the NHS to transfer money to individuals rather than to commissioners or providers. However, to make PHBs as inclusive as possible, it has been necessary to develop a continuum of options for how individuals can manage the money allocated to them rather than rely only on direct payments. The continuum allows PHB holders to exercise the same level of choice over how their needs are met, but with differing levels of responsibility for day-to-day money management. There are three broad options for how individuals can manage their PHB. They can take it as a 'direct payment' – a cash payment into their bank account; it can be managed by a third party; or it can continue to be held by commissioners as a notional or virtual budget. At present the legislative authority to offer a direct payment only covers pilot sites, but the Department of Health is extending the reach of the legislation to allow all CCGs to offer them (DH, 2013). However, it is important to remember that PHBs can be offered as notional or managed budgets without any further legislative changes and, therefore, CCGs that want to proceed with implementation do not need to delay.

This chapter discusses each of the money management options in turn before looking at the way in which PHBs are monitored and how commissioners judge whether or not they are effective. According to the Department of Health, having choice over money management is an essential part of a PHB, and whichever option a budget holder chooses, it is critical that they can exercise as much control as they choose over how and when the money is used (Fitzgerald et al, 2012a).

The three money management options

It is critical that all three money management options are available in each local area to give individuals maximum choice and not restrict PHBs to those who are interested in taking on greater responsibility. Which option is most appropriate will depend on a range of factors: the PHB holder's confidence in taking on financial responsibility; the size and complexity of the PHB and care plan; the amount of family and peer support available to the PHB holder; the extent to which the care plan includes hiring staff; and other factors. PHB holders and commissioners must both agree to the chosen option.

Direct payments

If an individual chooses to take the PHB as a direct payment, this has to be paid into a separate bank account, unless it is a one-off payment, in which case it can be paid into a personal bank account. Recurring direct payments can be paid into a bank account already set up for a social care direct payment. Individuals must have the capacity to consent to receive a direct payment or they must have a nominated representative and their care plan must include a named care coordinator. Those who are under the jurisdiction of the criminal justice system are legally unable to receive a direct payment but can still have a managed PHB (DH, 2010a).

Most PHB holders opt for a direct payment because they want to maximise choice and control. With a direct payment, the individual is truly the customer and has the flexibility to negotiate with providers and run their budget exactly as they choose. However, a direct payment brings with it responsibility. PHB holders are responsible for ensuring that clinical requirements are met, for example, that staff receive appropriate training and providers are professionally licensed where this applies. Individuals are also financially responsible and must be able to demonstrate that they have spent their direct payment according to their care plan.

Perhaps the greatest responsibility that comes with accepting a direct payment is that the PHB holder becomes an employer if they choose to hire staff as part of their care plan. They have to comply with the legal duties of being an employer, such as paying tax and National Insurance for staff, providing statutory benefits and dealing with disciplinary issues if they arise. Unions have raised concern about the extent to which direct payments in health and social care may erode security for direct care staff if individuals are not aware of the full extent of their responsibilities and are not properly supported to act as responsible employers (Unison, 2009).

To address these issues, it is critical that anyone choosing to have a direct payment has access to a direct payment support service. These are already in place in some areas because they provide support to social care direct payment holders, but coverage is patchy. Direct payment support services help budget holders with pay roll and financial management and can advise on employer responsibilities. They can be commissioned directly by the NHS and provided free of charge to PHB holders or they can be purchased directly by PHB holders who need the additional support.

The majority of direct payment support services are provided by small, third sector organisations that operate in a single local authority area. There are only a few organisations with regional or national reach, for example, Penderels Trust (www.penderelstrust.org.uk) and the Rowan Organisation (www.therowan.org). As the scale of PHBs grows and adds to personal budgets in social care, there may be a need for larger, more efficient providers to enter the market to boost capacity by partnering with local third sector organisations (Bennett and Stockton, 2011).

Financial management in the US

In the US Medicaid programme, individual budget programmes for home and community-based services are not authorised to pay money directly into individual bank accounts. This has led to the growth of financial management entities that hold and administer the money on behalf of individuals, in a similar way to a direct payments support service.

PCG Public Partnerships, LLC (PPL) is the largest provider of financial, administrative and support platforms for individual budgets in the US Medicaid programme, and has been providing support services since 1999. PPL's technological infrastructure enables individuals of all ages to serve as employers of personal assistants, to develop and manage individual budgets and to purchase the goods and services needed to live in their own homes. It also allows public authorities to offer real choice and control to individuals who do not wish to directly manage funds, and supports public authorities to retain oversight and budgetary control of self-directed programmes that is a priority for Medicaid.

PPL operates in 22 states in the US and has contracts with over 40 different government and health insurance organisations. It supports more than 42,000 individual budget holders, more than 44,000 directly hired personal assistants and is involved in US$530 million worth of transactions linked to individual care plans.

Source: www.publicpartnerships.com

Third party managed budgets

Under the third party option, the PHB holder nominates an organisation to receive the money on their behalf. Third parties can take many forms. They can be independent user trusts set up specifically to manage a PHB on someone's behalf, existing user-led organisations, care agencies or other provider organisations that offer third party management as an additional service. Since third party management involves a contract between the NHS and the third party, commissioners may specify the kind of organisation that is acceptable as a third party. For example, for very large PHBs with complex care plans, commissioners in the past have insisted that a third party be regulated by the CQC. An administration fee from the PHB goes to the third party to pay for its services.

The most significant difference between third party management and a direct payment is that, under third party management, the third party, not the individual, acts as the employer of record. This means that employment responsibility rests with the third party and the third party deals with day-to-day financial management, and can provide substantial back-up and advice in dealing with recruitment and any staffing issues that may arise. The third party can also help with support planning, accessing training, developing staff competencies and managing risk, particularly if the third party has a clinical background as a provider organisation. They may even provide information and advice about the condition itself. Similar models exist in other countries, for example, the agency with choice model of self-direction in the US that allows individuals to choose their staff without having to act as an employer (Murphy et al, 2012).

Individuals with large CHC PHBs often prefer to work with a third party given the size and complexity of the budget. However, there can be tensions with third parties as to who is in charge. As the Department of Health guidance states, individuals who use a third party should have as much control over how the money in their PHB is used as those who take a direct payment. Therefore, third parties must allow the family to be in control of the day-to-day management of the PHB, to hire and supervise the staff they want, to set pay rates and to judge whether staff have met certain competencies. The third party is there to provide support and advice, for example, by conducting interviews with the family, rather than to run things for the family. If the third party's risk management policies prevent the family from having day-to-day control, the arrangement is unlikely to give the family an adequate sense of choice and control (Fitzgerald et al, 2012).

The lack of availability of high quality third party organisations is a barrier to choice for many PHB holders who may prefer third party management over a direct payment. Market development is discussed further in Section 3. As well as focusing on provider development to ensure that PHB holders have adequate service options, commissioners will need to play an active role in expanding the market for the kinds of infrastructure discussed in this section, including third party management, direct payments support services and independent brokerage.

Notional or virtual budgets

The third option is for the management of the PHB to remain with commissioners in the form of a notional or virtual budget. With this option, commissioners continue to make the purchases, but individuals should know how much is in their budget before they start to plan, and should have the same flexibility to design their care plan and hire staff as they would under the other two options. One of the principle reasons for providing a notional budget is if money is tied up in block contracts with existing providers and cannot be transferred to the individual or to a third party. Under this scenario, individual service funds can be used to transition from block purchasing to individualised funding. An individual service fund sits within a block contract with a provider but is designated to a particular individual, and can be used as the individual chooses. In some senses, the provider acts as a third party but the money is not transferred to the provider in the form of a PHB. A PHB is carved out of an existing, larger contract (Fitzgerald et al, 2012a). Other decommissioning strategies that free up funds from existing services to provide PHBs are discussed in Chapter 10.

The challenge with notional budgets for the NHS is to ensure that they offer real choice and control. Pilot sites did find it cumbersome to purchase non-traditional goods and services on behalf of PHB holders through standard NHS procurement processes, often leading to significant delays. We know from experience in social care that notional budgets in many local authorities have been implemented in a restrictive way, although that does not have to be the case. Budget holders are limited to providers where there is already a contract in place with the council. Even where the council has moved out of block purchasing and operates spot purchasing under a framework contract, individuals may still be restricted to pre-qualified providers who are part of the framework contract. Individuals are not able to hire their own staff and cannot purchase non-traditional goods and services (Routledge and Lewis, 2011).There may be a need to provide notional budgets as a transition out of block contracts in the NHS. In the longer term, the emphasis should be on developing third parties to ensure that PHB holders who do not want a direct payment have a real alternative.

Monitoring personal health budgets

One of the most common concerns about PHBs is that individuals will use their budgets fraudulently, or allow their budgets to be abused. Drawing on evidence from personal budgets in social care that are far more widely used internationally, there is little evidence of fraud and abuse (Fox, 2012). In general, budget holders pursue value for money, negotiating prices with providers, maximise the use of free resources and only use what is required to meet their needs (Forder et al, 2012). Furthermore, money is transferred to individuals in increments, reducing the risk of significant overspending and increasing the likelihood that problems will be spotted before they get too serious. Where commissioners have real concerns about an individual's ability to manage a PHB prudently, a direct payment can be refused and third party management put in place.

Commissioners have a responsibility to monitor whether funds are being used as set out in an individual's care plan. Individuals or third parties on their behalf need to submit time sheets and receipts on a regular basis to demonstrate that money has been used correctly. As PHBs expand, commissioners may consider switching to an audit-based system, as has happened in social care, rather than monitoring every purchase. Individuals keep documentation to justify purchases, but only a sample of PHB holders are monitored at any one time. In some local areas, the NHS and social care have started to use pre-loaded payment cards as a way of transferring direct payments to individuals. The payment cards are linked to a central account, and every item of spending can be seen by commissioners without individuals having to submit any paperwork. This makes monitoring more streamline and efficient.

The Kent card

The Kent card is a pre-paid Visa card that was introduced by Kent County Council in conjunction with the Royal Bank of Scotland for social care direct payments and extended to PHBs as part of the pilot programme. Many local authorities are now using pre-paid cards because they reduce the risk of fraud and make it far easier to track spending. They are also being used internationally, for example, by the self-directed mental health pilots in Texas and Pennsylvania, discussed in Section 1. Budget holders can choose to have a Kent card rather than having their direct payment paid into a bank account. The direct payment is automatically transferred onto the card by Kent County Council each month. As with all direct payments, the card must only be used to purchase items that have been authorised as part of the individual's care plan, and individuals are expected to keep receipts for proof of purchase. The cards can be set up to allow cash payments if necessary and, unlike a credit or debit card, will not allow individuals to spend more than what is held on the card. Card holders receive a statement of their purchases every month, and this can also be seen by commissioners. Individuals do not need to set up a bank account to have a Kent card and, therefore, the option is open to all.

Source: Royal Bank of Scotland and Kent County Council, *Kent card holder guide: Making the most of your card* (https://shareweb.kent.gov.uk/Documents/adult-Social-Services/direct-payments/kent-card-holder-guide.pdf)

While financial monitoring attracts media attention, a far more important aspect of monitoring is the assessment of whether or not PHBs make a difference to people's health and wellbeing. This sort of assessment should be the focus of the review process for PHBs – the seventh step in the process outlined in Chapter 6. This necessitates a mind shift from a focus on what people purchase and the unusual items they buy to assessing the outcomes they manage to achieve with what they buy. Do PHB holders achieve the outcomes identified in their care plans, such as returning to work, rebuilding relationships with family members and using fewer emergency services? Table 9.1 presents a selection of purchases made in the Northamptonshire pilot for mental health and the planned outcomes they were used to achieve. It is important that outcomes are measurable to allow proper assessment of whether or not they have been met. While each individual will have different goals, it is possible to look at the overall effectiveness of PHBs by considering the extent to which individuals make progress towards or meet their goals.

The frequency with which a PHB will be reviewed should be set out in a person's care plan. An annual review is the minimum, and in many cases, can be built into the regular cycle of reviews rather than being separate for PHBs. However, individuals should feel free to agree a different pattern of review with their care coordinator, particularly in the early days of having a PHB. More frequent reviews can take place over email or telephone rather than in person. If an individual's needs change substantially, a review should be triggered immediately. This may result in the need for a reassessment to adjust the value of an individual's PHB rather than simply making changes to the care plan (Brewis et al, 2012).

Table 9.1: Selected outcomes and purchases from the Northamptonshire PHB pilot for mental health, February 2012

Category	Non-traditional purchase	Outcomes
IT equipment	PDA 'tablet' organiser Sat Nav	To help me keep in touch with others, organise my diary and access information To feel in control, competent, useful and maintain my independence
Therapies	Physiotherapy Massage/Indian head massage	Reduce stiffness and protective tension due to pain – a side-effect of my SSRI anti-depressant To compliment occupational therapy, understanding stress and anxiety and to have alternative ways to overcome stress
Education	Self-confidence course Microsoft Office	To feel safe and confident on my own so my wife will not have to be a 24/7 carer and improve my ability to engage in social activities To work and become part of society again. Long-term aim, to live on my own, independent from my family
Respite	Holiday with family Visiting family, travel costs	To re-establish a mother's relationship with her children – "be a good mum to my sons" My moods will be manageable, less reliance on current services and less chance of a relapse
Exercise	Shiatsu sessions Personal trainer	Weight reduction, control or reverse Diabetes type 2 diagnosis Increase strength and reduce pain

Source: Author's correspondence with PHB project manager in NHS Nene Clinical Commissioning Group, Northamptonshire

Section 2 has provided an overview of the investment in infrastructure needed to successfully implement PHBs. The implementer's checklist below provides a 10-point summary of the most important aspects of implementation. It is based on the experience of pilot sites in the national PHB programme. If implementers follow this checklist, it is highly likely that PHBs will have a positive impact on individuals and families and be cost-effective for the NHS. Section 3 turns to look at how PHBs fit within the wider NHS landscape and the challenge PHBs pose to NHS practice, clinical professionals and providers.

The implementer's checklist

1. Information about PHBs is available locally and there are clear guidelines about how PHBs work.
2. People know how much they have to spend upfront on their health and wellbeing.
3. Budgets and care plans address health and wellbeing, not just clinical treatment.
4. There is flexibility in how needs can be met and there are no menus that restrict choice.
5. Clinicians work with individuals and families as partners, respecting their expertise.
6. Support for budgets holders focuses on those who need it and is available on an ongoing basis, not just around the development of a care plan.
7. The entire PHB process is simple, transparent and designed to minimise bureaucracy.
8. Positive risk taking is encouraged and risks are documented and addressed in care plans.
9. Market development reflects the principles of co-production to ensure that PHB holders have adequate choice over support services and access to a diverse range of providers, including peers.
10. Reviews are conducted regularly in response to each individual's needs and are based on outcomes.

Sources: Alakeson (2012); Cattermole (2012c)

Section 3

Personal health budgets and organisational change in the NHS

TEN

Navigating the new landscape: personal health budgets and NHS reform

When it was first proposed that PHBs be piloted within the NHS, primary care trusts (PCTs) were responsible for commissioning services. Over the three years of the pilot, PCTs built up valuable knowledge and expertise about the best way to implement PHBs locally. However, when the Coalition government came into power in 2010, it proposed a sweeping round of structural reforms to the NHS that replaced PCTs with CCGs, alongside other far-reaching changes. As a result of these reforms, PHBs will be rolled out in a different commissioning environment from the one in which they were piloted. This may have its advantages: GPs spend the majority of their clinical practice seeing people with long-term conditions at all levels of complexity, and as lead commissioners within CCGs they may, therefore, be quicker to appreciate the benefits of a personalised approach. However, with CCGs only fully taking over commissioning responsibilities from PCTs in 2013, the challenge they face is to be ready for the roll-out of PHBs by April 2014.

Given the lack of stability in the wider NHS landscape, there is a risk that the momentum behind PHBs will wane as the deadline for roll-out approaches. Innovation that challenges established practice, as personalisation does, can be difficult to sustain in an uncertain, changing environment. Staff are distracted by job losses and new roles rather than focusing on improving the way in which they work with individuals who use services. A further distraction is the ongoing efficiency drive in the NHS. Latest estimates suggest that the NHS in England faces a funding gap of £14 billion between 2014/15 and 2021/22, even if funding for the NHS rises in line with GDP growth (Roberts et al, 2012). Bridging this gap will require a laser focus on efficiency savings, shifting attention away from PHBs. At the same time, the 2012 Health and Social Care Act that cemented the government's structural reforms in legislation undeniably presents opportunities for PHBs. Its guiding principle of 'nothing about me, without me' fits closely with the individual choice and control offered by PHBs (DH, 2012g). This chapter looks at the new landscape of the NHS and how this affects PHBs. The second half of the chapter focuses in detail on commissioning and the advantages and challenges that PHBs present for CCGs.

The new NHS landscape

The 2012 Health and Social Care Act created a set of new NHS organisations and swept away a series of others. Figure 10.1 shows how the new structures of the NHS relate to each other and to the public health responsibilities being taken over by local authorities. These new structures and their responsibilities will be described in turn. Other organisations have been created or their remit expanded as part of changes to the regulatory and performance management structures of the NHS. For example, Monitor has gained new powers as an economic regulator. These are not discussed in any detail in this chapter as they are less specifically relevant to PHBs, although highly relevant to the government's broader priorities for reform.

Figure 10.1: The new structures of the NHS

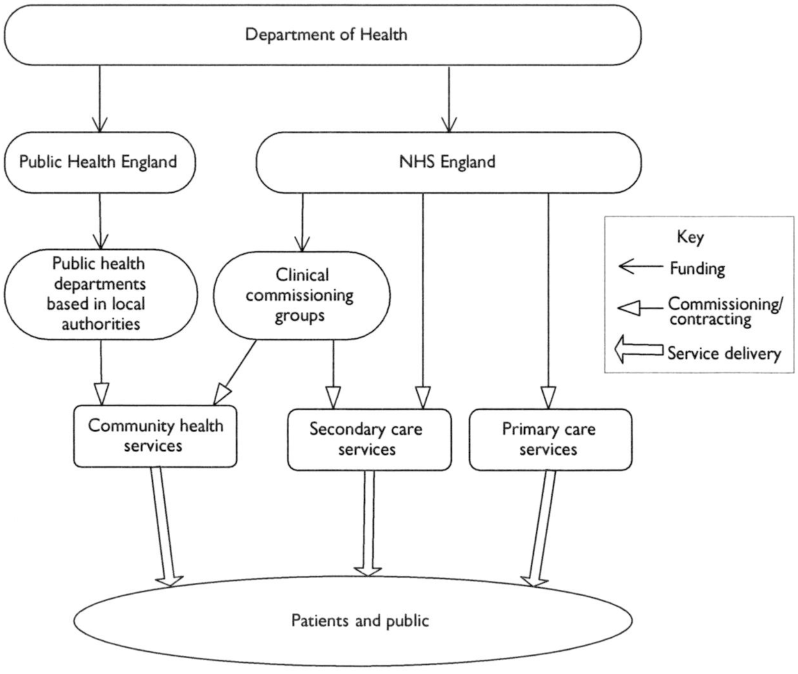

Source: Adapted from Holder and Thorlby (2012)

NHS England

NHS England was formally established in October 2012 as an independent, statutory body at arm's length from government (and was at the time called the NHS Commissioning Board). One of the central objectives of setting up NHS England was to take politicians out of the day-to-day running of the NHS. The Department of Health sets objective for the NHS in the form of a mandate that covers a three-year period. NHS England then holds CCGs responsible for the achievement of these objectives. NHS England sets the budget for each CCG and commissions specialised services, primary care services, offender healthcare and some services for the armed forces itself through 27 local area teams. Strategic health authorities that were previously responsible for the strategic direction of the NHS have been scrapped, and NHS England will instead have four regional arms.

Public Health England

The 2012 Act moved responsibility for public health from the NHS to a new body, Public Health England. The role of Public Health England is to protect and improve the health and wellbeing of the population and to reduce inequalities in health and wellbeing outcomes. It will also be responsible for commissioning substance misuse treatment and recovery services. Funding for public health will be allocated by Public Health England to directors of public health who will be based in local authorities.

Clinical commissioning groups

A total of 211 CCGs have replaced 152 PCTs as the main commissioning bodies within the NHS. CCGs are statutory bodies that cover a population of between 68,000 and one million people, with the median population size being 226,000, similar to the median PCT population of 228,000 (Naylor, 2012). CCGs will be responsible for commissioning the majority of services on behalf of their local population, including planned hospital care, rehabilitation, urgent and emergency care, most community health services and mental health and learning disability services. CCGs are clinically led and all GP practices have to belong to a CCG and provide primary care leadership to the commissioning process. CCGs will be supported by 23 commissioning support services that will work across several CCGs to provide organisational support such as IT services, human resource functions and data analysis.

Health and wellbeing boards

Health and wellbeing boards are not part of the new commissioning architecture of the NHS and are, therefore, not shown in Figure 10.1, but are an important feature of the new performance management system for the NHS. They are statutory bodies at the local authority level that bring together local commissioners from the NHS, public health and social care, elected representatives and members of the public. They have three main functions: to assess the needs of the local population through a joint strategic needs assessment process; to produce a local health and wellbeing strategy as the overarching framework for commissioning; and to promote greater integration and partnership between health and social care, including joint commissioning, integrated provision and pooled budgets where appropriate. Through this third function they may be instrumental in bringing social care personal budgets and PHBs into a single, integrated individual budget.

The new landscape and personal health budgets

The government's 2013-15 mandate to NHS England is unequivocal in demanding the NHS places greater emphasis on patients as partners in the management of long-term conditions, giving them greater choice, a more central role in decision making and valuing their experience of care on a par with safety and clinical effectiveness:

> The NHS Commissioning Board's [now NHS England's] objective is to ensure the NHS becomes dramatically better at involving patients and their carers, and empowering them to manage and make decisions about their own care and treatment. For all the hours that most people spend with a doctor or nurse, they spend thousands more looking after themselves or a loved one. (DH, 2012b, p 9)

To reflect this priority, the mandate includes objectives related to self-management and care planning. By 2015, NHS England must ensure that more people have developed the knowledge, skills and confidence to manage their own health and that everyone with a long-term condition is offered a personalised care plan that reflects their preferences and agreed decisions. The extension of PHBs is a further component of this drive to increase patient and carer empowerment, and much of the tone of the mandate's requirements in the context of long-term conditions reflects the thinking behind PHBs. It emphasises health and wellbeing and calls for care that is 'coordinated around the needs, convenience and choices of patients, their carers and families – rather than the interests of organisations that provide care'; 'centres on the person as a whole, rather than on specific conditions'; 'ensures people experience smooth transitions between care settings and organisations'; and 'empowers service users so that they are better equipped to manage their own care as far as they want and are able to' (DH, 2012b, pp 10-11).

The mandate creates an option for anyone who could benefit from a PHB to have access to one, with the government committed to starting from April 2014 with those who are eligible for NHS CHC and parents of children with special educational needs or disabilities, who will be able to ask for a personal budget based on a single assessment across health, social care and education (see Chapter 1 for further details). As discussed, implementation of PHBs will now be taken up by CCGs, although local authorities will have a lead role in the context of substance misuse where commissioning responsibility sits with Public Health England and directors of public health. The mandate's commitment to PHBs is reflected in NHS England's planning guidance to commissioners which highlights PHBs together with personalised care planning as priorities for the management of long-term conditions (NHS Commissioning Board, 2012). This builds on an instruction to commissioners in the 2012/13 NHS Operating Framework to consider the local implementation of PHBs as part of the transition of commissioning responsibilities from PCTs to CCGs (DH, 2011c).

Personal health budgets and commissioning

In Section 2, we looked at how to implement PHBs – the infrastructure that was necessary to make them work locally. This chapter considers what PHBs can offer commissioners. With CCGs under pressure to improve quality and value for money in the NHS, where can PHBs help (Imison, 2011)?

- Around 15 million people in England have one or more long-term conditions. They are among the most frequent users of healthcare services, but between 70 and 80 per cent of this group can be supported to manage their own condition. PHBs can play an important role in self-management and in supporting people to live well with an ongoing condition, as discussed in detail in Chapter 4. This is an area where the NHS, with its traditional focus on a clinical cure, has traditionally had less to offer. In supporting self-management, PHBs can help commissioners to deliver better health and wellbeing outcomes, to reduce unplanned hospital admissions and to improve people's experience of care. As the national evaluation demonstrates, PHB are a cost-effective route to improving care-related quality of life for individuals with long-term conditions (Forder et al, 2012).

- Greater secondary prevention for those with long-term conditions could substantially improve health outcomes and potentially lower costs by reducing the development of complications and slowing the progression of long-term conditions. PHBs have an important contribution to make to secondary prevention by supporting individuals to address their weight and other lifestyle issues in alternative ways to those traditionally offered by the NHS. As Tables 2.1 and 5.3 illustrate, bikes, gym memberships and weight loss classes have all been popular uses of PHBs with positive health effects.

- Reducing the amount of unplanned hospital activity related to conditions that can be managed in the community is an important dimension of improving the health of individuals with long-term conditions, improving efficiency and reducing the distress of emergency situations for individuals. The national evaluation has demonstrated a significant reduction in inpatient costs for PHB holders compared to the control group, and lower total costs for those with high value PHBs, indicating that real reductions in service use are achievable through PHBs (Forder et al, 2012).

- Many people with long-term physical health conditions also have mental health problems, often as a result of the limitations that their physical health problems place on their life. These co-morbidities make people less responsive to treatment and also add to the costs of care. For example, the total cost to the health service of each person with diabetes and co-morbid depression is 4.5 times greater than the cost for a person with diabetes alone (National Collaborating Centre for Mental Health, 2010). The national evaluation of PHBs has highlighted the potential of PHBs to provide more holistic care for those with mental health and physical health problems. Those who received a PHB for a physical health problem also reported improvements in their mental health and vice versa (Davidson et al, 2012, p 6).

- For those with highly complex conditions, care coordination can be a major challenge, and poorly coordinated care can significantly reduce people's quality of life. In the context of CHC, PHBs have demonstrated that they can improve the quality and coordination of complex care packages by putting individuals and families in control. Families report significant improvements in the reliability and continuity of care when they are able to hire their own teams who are specifically chosen to meet the health and wider wellbeing needs of the PHB holder and their family.

- National research indicates that 50 per cent of the population would choose to die at home. However, in 2008, only 20 per cent died at home compared to 55 per cent who died in hospital. PHBs have already supported some individuals who wanted to die at home to do so. There are challenges, notably the speed with which a budget needs to be put in place to be useful at the end of life. However, PHBs and the person-centred planning that is integral to them, do provide a tool to transform end of life care in line with people's wishes. If the care planning can be done in advance, the identified plan can quickly be put in place once an individual reaches the final stages of life (Alakeson and Duffy, 2011).

- Finally, as commissioning moves in the direction of greater integration between health and social care, PHBs provide a tool to support integration, with significant potential for reductions in the use of social care as well as NHS services. The PHB evaluation recommends that 'personal health budgets should be considered as a vehicle to promote greater service integration' (Forder et al, 2012, p 168). Several local areas are experimenting with the 'dual carriageway approach' to integrating personal budgets and PHBs discussed in Chapter 1 (Bennett and Stockton, 2012). In addition, there are opportunities for wider savings to government as people become less isolated and less dependent on public services, see their quality of life improve and become more actively involved in their communities and in employment.

Personal health budgets and the challenges for commissioners

As well as offering significant opportunities for commissioners, PHBs present a set of challenges that have not been addressed by the pilot programme. To date, the scale of PHBs in each local area has barely exceeded 100 people. As a result, it has been possible to introduce PHBs and continue to run existing systems side by side. The double running costs that have been incurred have not been significant enough for commissioners to need to release money from existing provider contracts. Furthermore, the first phase of the roll-out of PHBs will focus on CHC that is largely commissioned on a bespoke, individual basis. This is not to say that the culture change required in CHC will not be significant, but it will affect clinical practice more than the commissioning process.

The extension of PHBs to other long-term conditions, however, will present a much tougher challenge for commissioners, particularly in community services where block contracts are still the norm. Money will have to be released from existing provider contracts to free up resources for PHBs and make real choice possible for individuals. However, this process of decommissioning needs to be undertaken at a pace that allows providers the chance to adapt so that the market does not actually shrink, leaving individuals with fewer choices than before. At the same time, commissioners will have to stimulate the market to create alternatives for PHB holders. Many of these challenges have already been faced with the introduction of personal budgets in social care, and CCGs can learn much from the experience of local authorities, discussed in Section 1. We turn to the role of commissioners in market development later in this section. The rest of this chapter focuses on the challenge of decommissioning.

Decommissioning is a central priority within the NHS and is a prerequisite for a range of reforms. Without the ability for money to follow the choices made by individuals, there are barriers to opening up the provider market to any qualified provider as much as there are to the roll-out of PHBs. As such, wider momentum behind decommissioning should support PHBs. First and foremost, there is a need to establish the individual cost of services that are currently purchased on a block basis. Second, commissioners will need to work with a range of transition strategies to support providers to move away from block purchasing to more flexible arrangements such as framework contracts and spot purchasing while remaining sustainable in the marketplace.

In Chapter 9 we discussed individual service funds as a means of creating a degree of personalisation within a block contract. In addition, commissioners can adopt the following approaches to shifting resources out of block contracts over time (Audit Commission, 2012):

• Commissioners can phase in PHBs by keeping the total contract value with a provider the same but introduce a percentage of the contract that must be delivered as PHBs. This percentage can increase year on year to allow providers to unbundle their services and develop unit costings over time. This will put providers on a stronger footing to eventually adjust to not having any guaranteed income.

- Commissioners can reduce the total contract size for providers in line with the choices of PHB holders. If individuals continue to choose services from NHS providers, these can be commissioned directly as would have been done in the past. Other services will be purchased by individuals or third parties from outside the NHS. If the services provided by the NHS are not popular with PHB holders, traditional providers will see their income fall year on year.
- Commissioners can recoup money from providers on the basis of the choices that individuals make. This is the approach NHS Northamptonshire will operate from April 2013 for mental health, taking the PbR cluster tariffs discussed in Chapter 7 as a starting point. Commissioners will pay the NHS provider the cluster cost for the person following a cluster assessment or review. This will form that person's indicative budget. The individual will then work with the care coordinator and broker to write a personal plan and choose the services they want to meet their outcomes. The services provided by the NHS will be clearly priced and the broker, who will not be employed by the NHS provider, can act as a neutral advocate for the person. The costs of the services and supports that are not provided by the NHS provider will be released to the individual as a direct payment or to a third party.
- Commissioners can also use the Commissioning for Quality and Innovation (CQUIN) payment framework as a tool to stimulate changes towards personalisation among providers. The framework is based on locally set goals between commissioner and provider, and these can be directly linked to PHBs. For example, in 2009/10 Devon and Torbay PCT used its CQUIN framework to increase the number of people receiving mental health services from Devon Partnership Trust who took up a personal budget or PHB (Devon Partnership NHS Trust, 2011).

PHBs represent a significant change of role for commissioners in certain areas of the NHS. Individuals become the direct purchasers of services and commissioners take on the role of market shaping, working more closely than before with individuals, families and providers, as discussed later in Chapter 12. PHBs also present significant changes for clinical professionals as they shift from a position of expert authority to a partnership based on two sources of expertise. The implications and opportunities for clinicians are discussed in the next chapter.

ELEVEN

Doctor does not know best: a changing role for clinical professionals

We have already discussed how PHBs are a new tool for creating a more equal relationship between individuals and clinical professionals in which each contributes their own expertise in a genuine process of co-production. For occupational therapists and social workers familiar with self-directed support in social care, the change in working practice that PHBs require is not dramatic. For the majority of clinical staff in the NHS, however, PHBs represent a fundamentally different way of working from the way in which they were trained and traditionally practice. Care coordinators working in CHC in Manchester described the change in practice required to work with PHBs as at least an eight if not a ten out of ten, where ten represents a complete culture change.

The first dimension of that culture change is that PHBs start with the individual and balance what is important to that individual with what is important for their health. Traditional clinical practice starts with symptoms and diagnosis and rarely gets to know the mother, employee or music lover in the background. Pat Deegan eloquently describes how her diagnosis of schizophrenia quickly became her identity:

> And that diagnosis took on what I call a master status in terms of my identity. The fact that I was Pat, that there were many aspects to who I was as a person became absolutely irrelevant. Once I held this label, this diagnosis, what mattered was that I was a 'schizophrenic'. (Deegan, 2008)

Second, working in partnership with individuals requires clinicians to make decisions with, rather than for, people. This demands the skills of a health coach such as motivational interviewing and decision support counselling rather than conventional consultation skills, as Dr Greg Rogers discusses in his clinician's viewpoint on page 98 (Bennett et al, 2010). Third, PHBs start with an indicative budget and developing a care plan involves knowing how much different options cost. Few clinicians have experience of talking about money in their clinical practice, and many feel uncomfortable doing so. Finally, PHBs change the composition of the workforce, with independent support brokers and peers taking over roles previously performed by clinicians, creating fears about job losses and a tendency to defend the status quo.

Despite these challenges, clinicians with experience of working with PHBs report largely positive views. PHBs have given them something to offer those for whom they had run out of solutions. As one GP involved in the pilot programme commented, 'if we go on delivering the same services as we have done in the past, we're going to get the same outcomes and most people would accept that those aren't satisfactory' (Nene CCG, 2012). PHBs have allowed clinicians to work differently with people, often in ways that are closer to their original motivation for joining the NHS. As Sarah, an occupational therapist, puts it in her clinician's viewpoint on page 130, PHBs involve a 'freer, more personal way of working'. PHBs have even reduced the workload for some clinicians. For example, the CHC team in Oxfordshire found that care packages did not break down as often with PHBs as with traditional agencies, which meant that they had to deal with fewer crisis situations and out-of-hours calls (Reynolds, 2012).

Professional clinical bodies have also highlighted the opportunities that PHBs present. In its 2012 position statement on PHBs, the Royal College of General Practitioners identified four areas of opportunity: PHBs could increase the focus on care planning and stimulate shared decision making; they could provide opportunities for patients to access services provided by the voluntary sector that were better tailored to their needs; they could give patients greater control and flexibility over who provides their care and how and when it is delivered; and they could facilitate integration of services for patients with multiple and complex conditions, including integration between health and social care (Mathers et al, 2012). Similarly, in a policy paper in 2011, the Royal College of Nursing acknowledged the merits of PHBs as one tool to deliver more personalised care (Policy and International Department, 2011).

However, professional resistance to PHBs remains strong, and it is a concern that many clinicians feel poorly informed. In a small survey of doctors conducted in 2012, the British Medical Association found that 72 per cent felt not very well or not at all informed about the introduction of PHBs. Only a fifth of doctors surveyed felt that PHBs would be effective in putting patients in control of their care and 40 per cent did not support the use of PHBs to purchase goods and services outside the NHS (BMA, 2012). Similarly, a survey of over 600 clinical staff working in mental health found that 57 per cent of respondents knew little or nothing about PHBs and only 15 per cent felt that they knew a lot. Awareness of PHBs was highest among community psychiatric nurses and lowest among psychiatrists and psychologists (NMHDU, 2011a). Given their resistance to PHBs, it is common for clinicians to think that the NHS already offers individuals adequate choice and control or that improvements to existing initiatives such as care planning and shared decision making will make enough of a difference to people's health and wellbeing to make PHBs redundant. For example, 56 per cent of mental health staff were satisfied with the level of involvement that individuals had in their care, despite ongoing evidence from service users to the contrary (NMHDU, 2011a; BMA, 2012).

Building understanding of PHBs among clinicians will require ongoing training to be provided as part of the expansion of PHBs. This should include opportunities for clinicians to hear from PHB holders who are best placed to explain the difference PHBs can make to health and wellbeing. In addition, there are four objections to PHBs commonly raised by clinicians: PHBs do not respect evidence-based practice; they threaten clinical quality; increase risk; and potentially make it harder to control costs in the NHS. These concerns are understandable but can be addressed. The rest of this chapter considers each in turn.

Evidence-based care and personal health budgets

One of the central objections of clinicians to PHBs relates to evidence. This has two dimensions to it. The first is that there is inadequate evidence of the positive impact of PHBs, particularly evidence related to clinical outcomes. Among mental health staff, 53 per cent felt that there was inadequate evidence that choices made with a PHB would improve health outcomes (NMHDU, 2011a). The evidence base for PHBs, including the results from the national evaluation that demonstrated the positive impact of PHB, is discussed at length in Section 1.

The second dimension is that PHBs allow individuals to use NHS funding for goods and services that are not supported by evidence. This goes against the general principle of evidence-based care that underpins the NHS and is reinforced by NICE's work. The following view of a GP is typical:

> Yes there is choice, but we are still accountable for public money and therefore if you're going to ask for something non-evidence based it's not going to be reasonable. There is financial constraint and therefore we have to be even more aware of the fact that what we are going to spend our

money on is going to produce the goods ... we shouldn't be giving them things where there isn't evidence. This isn't going to give them good health outcomes. (quoted in NMHDU, 2011a, p 14)

When it comes to the tension between individual choice and evidence-based practice, the concerns of practitioners are easily understood given their clinical training. However, it is equally important to recognise the limitations of current evidence-based practice (Glasby, 2011a). First, clinical evidence is based on population averages and, therefore, can never hold true for every individual. There are instances when the recommended clinical treatment will not work for a particular individual and a new approach will be needed that PHBs can support. The Royal College of General Practitioners (RCGP) acknowledges this in its 2012 position statement: 'The RCGP accepts that certain treatments traditionally prescribed by the NHS do not work for some individuals and that, conversely, some treatments not traditionally prescribed by the NHS may be effective in improving health outcomes in certain cases' (Mathers et al, 2012, p 9). For example, Tom, who took part in the PHB pilot in Dorset, was able to return to work six months earlier than expected after a brain haemorrhage left him paralysed on his left side. By returning home rather than staying in hospital and using daily activities on the family's farm as rehabilitation as well as a personal trainer, fly fishing and swimming, Tom's recovery has been faster than his consultant could have expected (DH, 2012h).

Second, recommended clinical practice does not adequately recognise the added dimension of individual engagement that can make a real difference to outcomes (Hibbard et al, 2004). Take a person with depression – if they cannot establish a good rapport with their therapist and are not positive about the difference therapy could make, the treatment is unlikely to be successful, regardless of clinical guidelines. The engagement of individuals in the PHB process makes it more likely that their choices will lead to improvements.

Third, the current clinical evidence base tells us little about how to achieve the wider life outcomes that individuals care about most, such as getting a job or being a good parent. Filling this gap will require the development of a new evidence base generated through a process of co-production between the professional expertise of clinicians and the lived experience of service users. PHBs have an important contribution to make to the development of this evidence base (Alakeson and Perkins, 2012).

Clinical quality

There are concerns that if individuals are allowed to choose their own providers, they will receive lower quality care than is currently available through commissioned services.

> GPs and commissioners cannot guarantee the quality of services provided through personal health budgets, and patients may not have the knowledge to judge good quality services from poor-quality services. Although some service providers may be registered with the Care Quality Commission (CQC), where a patient uses an individual budget to arrange his or her own personal or nursing care without agency involvement, this service is exempt from the requirements for CQC registration. In addition, most complementary and alternative therapies are outside the scope of CQC regulation. (Mathers et al, 2012, p 10)

The quality of care delivered through a PHB can be ensured in several ways. First, if individuals access clinical care such as physiotherapy or counselling, commissioners can stipulate that only an appropriately qualified professional can deliver care. Second, where individuals are hiring their own personal assistants, PHBs should include funding for training, as highlighted in Chapter 7 to ensure that all staff meet appropriate standards. Third, as discussed in Chapter 9, individuals can receive their PHB through a third party organisation that can provide guidance, training and support for contingencies. Furthermore, as we saw in the discussion of evidence in Section 1, in contrast to the expectations of clinicians, several international studies find that in general, PHB holders report improvements in the quality of care they receive (Glendinning et al, 2008; Norris et al, 2010). PHB holders who hire their own staff report far greater reliability and continuity of care compared to care provided by agencies, particularly when they can set their own pay rates and create incentives for staff to stay with them for longer.

In many ways, the challenge PHBs pose to assessments of clinical quality is similar to the one they pose to the established clinical evidence base. Whose view of quality or evidence counts? PHBs put the individual's experience of care at the centre of how we judge quality and place less trust in paper qualifications. This is a challenge to traditional views of clinical quality that are only just starting to incorporate patient-reported outcomes. But in many ways individuals are best placed to judge quality because they have the most at stake. PHB holders have a stronger vested interest in ensuring that their staff are trained to meet their needs and keep them safe than commissioners who will never be on the receiving end of the care they purchase.

Managing risk

Many clinicians fear that PHBs place individuals at greater risk by allowing budget holders to make different decisions from those of professionals. For example, an individual with MS may choose to see a reflexologist to manage their pain rather than seeing a physiotherapist that could result in the condition worsening. They may choose to spend the vast majority of their budget on a holiday but the boost to their wellbeing does not last and they no longer have enough money to meet their needs for the rest of the year. Or a family member may put pressure on them to spend their budget in ways that benefit their family and not their health.

These are valid concerns, but these risks can be well managed through an effective PHB process. On the financial side, money is paid in instalments to prevent budget holders running out, and a third party can manage the budget if there are concerns about exploitation from family members. Care plans are also critical to managing risk, as discussed in Section 2. Clearly setting out the benefits and risks of individual choices can help protect clinicians in the case of an adverse event. Risks should be documented and the care plan should discuss how each risk will be managed.

Perhaps the most challenging aspect of risk management is the shift that PHBs require in how the NHS responds to risk. In making choices about how needs are met, PHBs do involve individuals taking greater responsibility for their care and taking well-managed, positive risks that can help them live a better life (Glasby, 2011b). For example, as well as his regular trips to the barbers, Martin, who we heard about in Chapter 2, chose to use his PHB to adapt his bike so that he could continue to get regular exercise and prevent his condition deteriorating. Inherent in his choice is the risk that he may fall off his bike and hurt himself, but given that this has never happened before, it is unlikely, and is far outweighed by the positive benefits for him of being able to continue cycling. Positive risk taking poses a challenge to the risk-averse culture of the NHS and its focus on safeguarding. All too often this results in an entirely negative view of risk that can limit people's opportunities to live well and be fulfilled. To encourage well managed, positive risk taking pilot sites have found it helpful to put in place a risk enablement panel. This is a multi-disciplinary panel that can be convened to discuss risk situations when frontline staff are not comfortable taking a decision alone (Carr, 2010). By sharing the responsibility for decision making among the group, the panel can facilitate more positive risk taking. In one local authority, the risk enablement panel for self-directed support is rarely convened, but it was essential at the beginning to reassure clinical staff unfamiliar with a personalised way of working (Eost-Telling, 2010).

Financial sustainability

The impact of PHBs on costs in the NHS is also an area of concern, particularly with GPs having greater financial incentives to manage spending through CCGs. Based on international experience and experience in social care, there are justifiable concerns that PHBs will increase demand for services and drive up costs by drawing people into the NHS who would not otherwise want an NHS service. This has been the case with the *Persoonsgebonden Budgets* programme in the Netherlands that experienced a ten-fold increase in demand for individual budgets between 2002 and 2010. The programme's eligibility and spending rules have since been tightened to better manage demand (White, 2011).

Another concern about financial sustainability is the extent to which the costs of providing services increases as a percentage of people leave the service to make different choices with their PHB. If enough people leave and the costs of providing the service do not fall proportionately because of fixed costs, for example, the service will be more expensive to provide for those who continue to use it. At a time of resource constraint, these issues of financial sustainability are rightly a concern for clinicians and commissioners. Some of the costs of PHBs are likely to be offset by lower healthcare use in other parts of the NHS, especially inpatient care. However, in the short term, the transition to greater use of PHBs will have to be carefully managed to minimise costs and not destabilise providers, as discussed in the previous chapter.

Beyond these specific issues, there is a broader, overarching concern among clinicians about the extent to which PHBs undermine the basic principles of the NHS: that care is free at the point of use and based on need, not locality or ability to pay. As discussed at the very beginning of this book, PHBs do not allow for top-ups of any kind. Care remains free at the point of use. However, there is a real risk, as discussed in Chapter 3, that a postcode lottery for PHBs will emerge because much of the decision making as to whether to offer PHBs, for whom and at what pace will remain in the hands of CCGs. Individuals who could benefit from a PHB may find that in their area, PHBs are not being offered for their condition. This must be guarded against as it is likely to exacerbate existing health inequalities.

Building greater support among clinicians for PHBs without undermining the core of the approach will be one of the central challenges of the next phase of PHBs. Imposing a menu of evidence-based practices from which budget holders can choose would reassure clinicians but reduce individual choice and, as we know, erode the positive impact of PHBs on quality of life and wellbeing (Forder et al, 2012). Working with PHB holders to engage clinicians in the positive benefits of PHBs will be important. Co-designing the marketplace with individuals and families will also be critical in response to the growing purchasing power of PHB holders. Market development is the subject of the next chapter.

An occupational therapist's view of personal health budgets

Sarah Perkins is an occupational therapist who took part in the PHB pilot for mental health in Northamptonshire. Before working with PHBs, Sarah had had some experience of working with self-directed support and personal budgets in social care and had found it really positive. The pilot in Northamptonshire focused on individuals who were receiving treatment and support from a community mental health team.

Interviewer: 'What reservations, if any, did you have before working with PHBs?'

Sarah: 'I had reservations about how to define health as opposed to social care needs in the context of mental health. What were the parameters of health need? And how would alternatives to traditional mental health services be justified and regulated? Would PHBs be helpful or detrimental?

'I had questions about whether PHBs were part of my remit as an occupational therapist and was unsure how my current working arrangement with clients would be quantified when setting a budget. I was also concerned about how time-consuming the administration of PHBs would be.'

Interviewer: 'How did the process of working with a PHB fit with your existing role? Did it create more of a workload?'

Sarah: 'PHBs fitted very well into my role. As an occupational therapist in mental health, my job focuses on working with someone to foster engagement in meaningful occupation, thinking about and identifying goals, developing or getting back into purposeful and productive roles. Identifying health needs through a PHB led to conversations about how these objectives could be achieved, with more thinking from the client and some thinking also from me, which is not far removed from conventional goal and intervention planning. I have wondered how other professions may find PHBs in terms of devising them with clients. The shift may be more difficult for clinical professions that are rooted in the medical model.

'In the end, if I were to make direct comparison to "ordinary" paperwork, there was little difference in compiling a PHB. The paperwork could be easily integrated with what the care programme approach requires in secondary care. Integrating the paperwork is essential. There is no time to do two lots.'

Interviewer: 'What did you find particularly positive about working with PHBs, for you as a clinician and for the people you work with?'

Sarah: 'Reflecting on the process, PHB planning gave me an opportunity to go back to the beginning with my client, to hear his story and gave him an opportunity to think about what exactly he felt in terms of what was important in life, what he wanted to change, redevelop or maintain. Sessions turned from focusing on problems to thinking about what would be helpful, and I got a sense that in the process he gained a sense of self-respect and reorientation to what was important for him. This in turn gave him the impetus to do other things in his life, so the PHB has in many ways been greater than the sum of its parts. There was a shift in perceived control from me to him, where I acted as more of an interpreter and mediator, sounding board and adviser. This was particularly important to the client, as mental health difficulties had stripped him of a sense of agency. It was a freer, more personal way of working.

'One of the most difficult aspects of working with a PHB is the budget allocation process and having to think about money and discuss spending with clients. This is not something that is normally part of a clinician's job and can feel uncomfortable for both sides. Some individuals feel that their PHB reflects the value that the NHS places on their life and are disappointed when it is low. When a PHB is seen as putting a price on someone's life, this needs to be handled very sensitively.'

Interviewer: 'Do you feel there are any remaining issues if PHBs are to be rolled out much further, beyond CHC?'

Sarah: 'How long does a PHB last? At what point is money reduced? I think there needs to be some thought given towards the provision of a maintenance budget, as in the scheme of things, people who have needed the resources of a secondary mental health service will in most instances remain in need of some support.

'Should the NHS pay for things that they haven't paid for up to now? I think this is a sticking point in most people's heads. I think you need to take a step back and ask the question of why we are looking towards alternatives. Often the resources and approaches available through the NHS are realistically not sufficient or effective.

'Also, it will be important to develop a process to ensure that independent resources are accountable and regulated in the case of personal assistants. However, if as was the case for me, the clinician remains integral to the process, then any concerns could be picked up and addressed promptly.'

Interviewer: 'Do you think that the reservations voiced by professional bodies will be dismantled as more people start to work with PHBs or is the culture change going to be very hard?'

Sarah: 'There is validity in the concerns of professional bodies such as the RCGP, although is the current situation ideal? The ease of adoption of change may be a generational one and may be profession specific. One important factor is whether the concept of PHBs is embraced by management.

'Current reservations could be addressed through greater publicity and training. Not knowing about PHBs can create doubts and misunderstandings. Training would give people a clear understanding of the structure and process of PHBs, some sense of their worth, and allow them to really dig deep to analyse the uncertainties and scrutinise the efficacy, reliability and quality of what's available now compared to what a PHB could offer.

'I wonder also how "popular" PHBs will be in the long run. Some reports have intimated that demand for PHBs could lead to more spending. In mental health, I believe there will be people who will not want to have to think about a PHB and will be happy with treatment as usual because it suits them. For other people, PHBs can help them feel more in control. Whether PHBs work for people is an individual thing that will largely depend on the character of the person.'

Source: Author's interview with Sarah Perkins, December 2012

TWELVE

Growing the market: bringing new providers into the NHS

PHBs necessitate a more diverse marketplace with a greater variety of providers to be able to cater effectively to the individual needs of budget holders. Experience from social care highlights the risk of offering personal budgets without focusing on market development. In some parts of the country, budget holders who had previously attended day programmes found themselves with few alternative ways of using their money once the day programme had closed. They had the resources to purchase alternatives, but the market had not responded to offer other choices (Needham, 2012). The US state of Michigan had a similar experience when it introduced a self-directed care programme for adults with mental health problems. Without first developing a workforce of certified peer specialists who could offer alternative services to individuals, there was little on offer for budget holders outside of the community mental health centres they were trying to leave.

As the national evaluation shows, PHB holders secured a different mix of services from that purchased by commissioners for the control group. For example, they purchased significantly more wellbeing services and used less hospital care. This meant that they relied on a different range of providers from traditional NHS commissioning. Based on the spending patterns of PHB holders in the pilot programme, the evaluation team estimates that around 12 per cent of the average value of a PHB in the pilot programme went to providers outside the NHS. On the basis of this estimate, the team recommends that 'policy makers should anticipate that the use of personal health budgets is likely to result in a higher level of expenditure going to "non-conventional" providers (for example, a greater use of non-NHS providers)' (Forder et al, 2012, pp 168-70). With significant amounts of money in search of new providers, it is vital that the market is adequately developed to respond (Glasby, 2012).

Through its Any Qualified Provider initiative, the government is seeking to introduce a greater diversity of private, independent and voluntary sector providers into community and mental health services so that individuals can receive care in ways that better suit their preferences. Any Qualified Provider is supported by the extension of PbR into mental health and community services, as discussed in Section 2. PbR provides a mechanism for money to follow individual choices rather than providers being commissioned through a block contract. While these reforms are controversial and have been resisted by many as the beginnings of privatisation within the NHS (Ramesh, 2012), they remain integral to the development of PHBs and the drive to personalise the NHS more widely.

Current commissioners also have an important role to play in market development. Even where they are not purchasing services directly, commissioners can work with existing providers and encourage new entrants as part of developing the flexibility and diversity that is needed to respond to PHB holders. This chapter sets out tools and strategies for commissioners to actively develop the marketplace, drawing on the experience of sites in the national pilot programme. It also considers what PHBs mean for traditional providers, and how they need to respond to remain viable in a more plural NHS.

Personal health budgets and provider innovation

One of the central motivations for introducing patient choice into the NHS was to improve provider performance driven by the pressure of competition. In part, because competition remains limited – outpatient provision by independent treatment centres accounted for only 3.5 per cent of all first appointments in 2010/11 (Kelly and Tetlow, 2012) – there is as yet little evidence of innovation in response to the needs of individuals among traditional NHS providers. For example, as part of the PHB pilot in Eastern and Coastal Kent, individuals like Yve (see page 83) could opt for a PHB instead of receiving psychological therapy from the local NHS trust. The vast majority of individuals who participated in the pilot chose to use their PHB for therapy, but from a private sector provider alongside some additional supports. From the perspective of PHB holders, private sector providers presented several advantages. Individuals could choose a therapist they had worked with before with whom they had a good rapport, improving the likelihood that the therapy would be successful. They could establish contact with the therapist by telephone or email in advance of their first session to establish a rapport before meeting in person, and change therapists if they did not feel that the relationship was positive. They could also vary the structure of the sessions to suit their needs, having shorter sessions over a greater number of weeks or sessions every other week over a longer period of time (Walton, 2012).

Although there is nothing to prevent NHS trusts offering similar levels of flexibility, they have not done so and continue to provide a standard offer for psychological therapies into which individuals have to fit. This is not a question of the evidence base about how therapy should be offered but more proof that trusts have not faced competitive pressures to innovate and attract individuals to their services.

PHBs have the potential to increase the pressure for innovation on existing providers, particularly if commissioners play an active role in encouraging market development and use contract changes to drive greater personalisation, as discussed in Chapter 10. As part the national pilot programme, NHS Southampton City offered PHBs for alcohol detoxification. The PHB support broker worked closely with individuals in the pilot to understand their needs and with providers to create new detox options. Alongside a traditional inpatient or residential detox, providers started to offer the option of a home detox, with individuals using part of their PHB to pay for a night sitter if they lived alone or to pay for childcare if they wanted to remain at home but would not be able to properly look after their children while undergoing treatment. Similarly, Dorset PCT introduced PHBs for people with an acquired brain injury as an alternative to the existing service that consists of a five-bed inpatient rehabilitation unit and a community rehabilitation team. For the three people who took up a PHB, rehabilitation was more successful and took less time than the traditional service. Commissioners are now working with existing providers to see whether they can change the traditional service to be more flexible and individually tailored (Cattermole, 2012d).

While a significant number of people will want to use their PHB outside the NHS and not purchase healthcare services as such, preferring gym memberships and computer equipment, a large number of PHB holders do not want to make dramatic changes to their care package. They simply want greater control over who provides the service, at what time and how it is provided. There are significant opportunities for traditional providers to respond to these budget holders if they can offer the kind of flexibility and innovation that is more common in the private and voluntary sectors (Bennett, 2012). If they resist innovation and continue to provide services as they always have, it is likely that they will lose ground to new entrants who are more willing to respond to individuals. Large domiciliary care providers are already having to make this transition in response to personal budgets in social care. For example, Dimensions, a national not-for-profit organisation providing support to people with learning disabilities and autism, has created staff profiles that include personal interests, and is offering service users the opportunity to work with someone who shares their interests and with whom they can develop a reciprocal relationship in line with the principles of co-production. In many ways, the innovation that is needed to respond to PHBs is part of the shift that providers should anyway make to offer a more responsive service to all service users, those who have PHB and those who do not.

Growing the market

Growing the market to meet the needs of individuals means that commissioners have to work more closely than before with budget holders and their families in order to understand what matters most to them; what they judge to be lacking in the current marketplace; and how they evaluate the performance of existing providers. This is where a local network of PHB users and their carers can be a real source of market intelligence (Bennett, 2012). We discussed the concept of co-production in Section 1. Co-production needs to be at the root of market development for PHBs. With it comes a focus not just on the creation of new services but also on the development of networks of support and other opportunities for reciprocity and community engagement (Boyle et al, 2010). This requires getting beyond user consultation to having people with lived experience designing, running and evaluating services and support in partnership with professionals (Stevens, 2011).

Encouraging the development of peer support in its many guises is central to market development for PHBs. Peer support helps people to feel less alone, fosters hope and images of possibility. It allows people to share experiences, understanding, ideas about dealing with challenges, and is of mutual benefit by enabling people to use their experience to help others facing similar challenges (Repper and Carter, 2010). A significant part of health services for long-term conditions is not technical treatment and does not require clinical professionals. In fact, there may be risks in using professionals to provide support in areas in which they are not expert, such as living with and rebuilding life with a long-term condition. 'Experts through lived experience' are better placed to play this role (Innovation Unit, 2012a).

Working with providers to develop a more mixed workforce with greater roles for peer providers will be critical. Support for user-led social enterprises and for PHB holders who want to start micro-enterprises to work with others in a similar situation can add particular value. As part of the development of personalisation for users of mental health services in Stockport, the Council and Pennine Care Trust with support from the charity, Nesta, are investing in a range of peer-led services and supports in order to create a fabric of alternatives for people with personal budgets who are looking to move out of secondary care. This includes a user-led crisis service, peer-led commissioning and peer-led assessments. Stockport's approach is rooted in the concept of co-production and the recognition that people with long-term conditions may need support but can continue to make a positive contribution to their peers and their community (Innovation Unit, 2012b).

The peoplehub: a network of personal health budget holders for personal health budget holders

The peoplehub was founded in 2012 by three carers of individuals with PHBs who have also been closely involved at the national level with the development of PHBs. The peoplehub describes its three objectives as follows:

- Giving a voice: we want to make sure that our voices count so we will seek out and actively listen to what people say about their experience of PHBs.
- Connect and empower: we believe that being connected to like-minded people in the development of PHBs will create confidence by showing people they are not on their own, and also provide a valuable opportunity to learn from each other.
- Influence developments: by influencing the development of PHBs we will ensure they stay true to purpose and reflect our learning.

Source: www.peoplehub.org.uk

Technology can be a significant enabler of market development through the creation of online directories and market places that can help budget holders, brokers and clinical professionals know what is available in their area. As discussed in Section 2, having good quality information is critical to the success of PHBs and online market places can empower budget holders to find the services and supports they need as well as providing a much needed shop window for micro-enterprises and self-employed providers. Shop4Support (www.shop4support.com) is an online market place for personal budget users in social care that allows budget holders to research and buy anything from a wheelchair to a nursing service. Shop4Support works with a broad range of local authorities to enable people to navigate the market place and access the services and supports they need. Online market places such as this could be expanded to cover a broader range of goods and services in response to PHB holders.

Registries of personal assistants can also be an important tool to grow the provider market. These are common in the US where they are run by state governments to provide better access to a pool of potential employees for individuals directing their own care and more consistent employment for workers. At their most basic, registries function as a directory, but they have also been developed to provide a direct matching service for individuals looking for personal assistants. For example, the Arkansas Direct Service Workers registry, which is managed by the Arkansas Department of Human Services, provides an internet-based matching service for individuals directing their own care and for individual providers (https://dhs.arkansas.gov/daas/dswregistry/default.aspx). The service provides budget holders with a list of potential personal assistants, including detailed information about their availability, expected pay, the services they provide and their contact information. Background checks are not completed before personal assistants are registered and remain the responsibility of the individual employer. The service is free for individuals looking to hire staff and for those registering to provide care.

Joining up self-direction and welfare to work in Colorado

As Colorado's self-direction program for adults with disabilities continues to expand, there is a growing need for personal assistants to work for those who gain control of their support services. The state has identified an overlap between the skills of welfare to work participants who are required to find a job and the skills required of personal assistants. It is, therefore, establishing a partnership between the Department of Works and the Department of Healthcare Financing and Policy. The Department of Works will carry out a screening process to identify those who have the right skills and abilities to work as personal assistants and will help them obtain the necessary training and complete the paperwork to be added to a registry of personal assistants. This partnership ensures that welfare to work participants have ready access to job opportunities in a growing sector, provides the Department of Works with an ongoing connection to a source of employment and gives individuals with a budget access to a pool of screened workers. A similar partnership between Work Programme providers and local authorities or CCGs in the UK could potentially support the needs of both parties as personalisation continues to expand.

Source: Author's correspondence with Public Partnerships, LLC that administers the self-direction program in Colorado

While PHBs may not be the preferred option for all service users, market development to support PHBs can benefit all users of the NHS. A more responsive service from traditional providers may help them to retain market share as the balance of commissioning shifts from block contracts to PHBs. But a more personalised service will also improve the offer to those who continue to use commissioned services. Furthermore, the choices that individuals make with their PHBs can help shape commissioning more broadly, ensuring that the all service users benefit from the market intelligence that PHBs generate.

Conclusion

A decade ago, the idea of the NHS allocating money directly to individuals to make choices about how best to meet their health needs was considered impossible. Direct payments in social care had been legal for only five years, and there were fierce objections to extending the approach into health, not least of which was that paying money to individuals was illegal. It is, therefore, remarkable that as of April 2014, PHBs will become an established feature of the NHS, starting with the 56,000 people eligible for NHS CHC. The speed of change has been impressive in a sector that is generally slow to adopt innovation.

PHBs have no doubt benefited from the cross-party support that personalisation as a strand of public service reform enjoys. This has meant that a pilot started under the previous Labour government has been picked up by the current Coalition one, and the decision to extend PHBs is unlikely to be reversed by any future government. But their success owes more to the evidence of their impact than to political favour. When subjected to a rigorous academic test through a national evaluation, PHBs passed with flying colours. They were shown to improve the quality of life and wellbeing of individuals with long-term conditions and disabilities, and to do so in a way that is cost-effective. A large part of that improvement stems not just from the way in which people choose to use their PHBs, but also from the very fact that they have that choice and control. This allows them to define their own outcomes and to use their lived experience and creativity alongside the expertise of clinicians to develop their own solutions.

We know from the stories in this book that PHBs can transform the lives of budget holders and their families. We have heard how much difference they have made to Stephen, Alex, Tom, Yve, Martin and Malcolm, and there are hundreds of others across the country who have benefited from the pilot programme. And they have the potential to benefit thousands more. However, that will all depend on how well they are implemented as they move beyond the pilot stage. The evaluation is unambiguous in its message: PHBs implemented in line with the policy of choice and control for individuals have the strongest impact. Too many restrictions on the choices individuals can make over how to spend and manage their money only lead to negative impacts.

Getting implementation right is now the challenge facing those involved in PHBs and the one to which this book responds. Based on the experience of the pilot sites and initiatives in other countries, the book's central messages for implementers are simple: establish clear guidelines early on for how PHBs work; allocate resources to cover health and wellbeing, not just clinical needs; provide individuals with adequate information, advice and support throughout the process; and ensure that people have the same choice and control regardless of which money management option they choose. Decisions about implementation will be specific to each local area and CCG, but respecting these basic ground rules when putting in place the infrastructure for PHBs will ensure a good start.

But the challenge that PHBs present to the NHS is not just the challenge of implementation; it is also the challenge of culture change. By demanding changes in NHS practice, PHBs require commissioners, clinicians and providers to work in new and different ways. This book highlights clear opportunities for those in the NHS who can adapt to working in partnership with individuals and families, can enable positive risk taking and are willing to learn from the evidence of lived experience. For commissioners, PHBs present opportunities to improve value for money in the management of long-term conditions at a time when NHS finances have never been tighter. This includes bringing together health and social care through the integration of personal budgets and PHBs. For clinicians, they can create a more personal way of working and offer new solutions where existing treatment options have failed. For providers, they offer new market opportunities in areas such as wellbeing services and open up the NHS to new types of providers such as peers, user-led organisations and micro-providers.

PHBs are at the vanguard of change towards a more patient-centred, personalised NHS, but their value is not simply in the transformation that they achieve for those who have a budget and those who work with them, but in the wider change they catalyse across the NHS. PHBs present an opportunity for the NHS to re-examine its purpose in light of today's health problems rather than those of half a century ago. As the burden of disease in the UK and other developed countries shifts more and more to long-term rather than acute health conditions, there is a growing case for the NHS to define its core purpose around the difference it can make to people's lives, not just the management of their condition. This is the focus that PHBs bring to the NHS. This new orientation would mean that the care offered by the NHS would be mindful of the contribution it could make to employment. NHS services would explicitly address social isolation and the availability of stable housing would be a legitimate question for the NHS to raise if this could make the biggest difference to someone's health. This is not to suggest that the NHS becomes a catch all-service, but more that we reconnect health to the rest of people's lives in the way that people themselves do.

Looking beyond the NHS, the expansion of personalisation is far from reaching its full potential. In some parts of public services where pilots have been tried, personalisation has yet to move from the fringes to the mainstream. Here consolidation is required to ensure that momentum is not lost. Even in adult social care, where personalisation is the central policy focus, implementation has gone awry in many places, and a renewed focus on achieving real choice and control for individuals is required. And for those who use more than one service, the integration of different funding streams into one individual budget remains an ongoing challenge. Only a minority of PHB holders who also received a social care personal budget were able to manage both through a single bank account. In some cases, administrative procedures that were set up for one budget were not considered adequate for the other, and separate systems had to be put in place. For some, there was considerable confusion as to what could be paid for with which budget (Forder et al, 2012).

Looking to the future, there are new areas of public services where personalisation could bring benefits. Commentators have argued that personalisation could be introduced into the criminal justice system as part of offender rehabilitation (Marsh and Fox, 2012). Given the successful use of individual budgets to resettle the long-term homeless and to move individuals with disabilities and mental health problems from long-stay institutions into the community, it seems clear that personalisation could play a role here. This could be focused around the development of a resettlement plan when in prison that could be put into action through an individual budget controlled by a lead professional rather than by individuals themselves.

Personalisation and welfare to work in the Netherlands

Personal reintegration budgets (*persoonsgebonden re-integratiebudget* or PRBs) are offered by 40 per cent of municipal authorities to provide jobseekers with employment support. An evaluation of PRBs in 20 municipalities found that the approach was more cost-effective at securing employment than traditional employment services.

A related approach called an IRO (*individuele reintegratie overeenkomst*) has been offered by the national employment agency since 2007, and is taken up by two thirds of jobseekers. The IRO model has also been found to increase an individual's chance of securing a job compared to traditional services, and is particularly cost-effective for disabled jobseekers.

Source: Tarr (2011)

International developments also provide insights into possible new areas for personalisation. In the Netherlands, individual budgets are used extensively and successfully in welfare to work (see above). UK experts have argued that 'personal welfare budgets' (PWBs) should be integrated into the Work Programme, the government's major new welfare to work initiative. The Centre for Economic and Social Inclusion estimates that the rate of job entry for those on Employment and Support Allowance who voluntarily participate in the scheme could increase from 51 per cent to 62 per cent, if PWBs achieved similar improvements to IROs in the Netherlands (Tarr, 2011).

Personalisation is often viewed as the soft option in public service reform. How is it possible to object to creating services that respond to their users? But personalisation is, in fact, a radical idea. By giving individuals control of the money that is currently spent on their behalf, the balance of power shifts away from professionals and managers of public services, towards individual users. This is a profound change and it is therefore not surprising that when personalisation is put into practice, it is often fiercely resisted. But as this book has illustrated, the example of PHBs shows that giving power to people is not just good for them in the sense that their wellbeing improves; it is good in the sense that their feeling of control over their own lives improves.

Public services exist to help people achieve their full potential. They provide services that are necessary and without which people would be bereft. A great deal of selfless work is done to achieve this objective. This book has shown that the most effective next step is to trust people with power, and offer them the support to shape a life for themselves. This is what personalisation is, in the end, all about, and this is what PHBs make possible in the NHS.

Epilogue

Jonathan's story

Jonathan has a tracheostomy and needs to carry a breathing unit with him at all times. He suffers from severe epilepsy which requires rectal medication. He has severe curvature of the spine, is double-jointed and has hypotonia. His health assessment describes him as having severe learning disabilities, severe behavioural problems, global development delays and no speech. He also has bilateral deafness and eczema.

In the three years immediately before leaving school Jonathan spent 150 days in hospital as a result of breathing problems. In the three years since leaving school he has spent only two nights in hospital, for elective dental treatments. This radical improvement in Jonathan's life was brought about by access to an integrated individual budget through the Personalised Transition programme at Talbot School in Sheffield. In the first three years, Jonathan's annual budget was about £70,000, split between health and education. The local authority continued to play a critical role in integrating the funding from different sources and enabling the family to manage it directly. This has allowed Jonathan's family to oversee the development of a personalised package of support based around flexibility, employment and on-the-job learning and to recruit personal assistants who are trained in how to support Jonathan's healthcare needs.

Jonathan's health needs are complex, but since getting his individual budget his life has been full and positive and his health has been getting better and better. For Katrina, Jonathan's mum, the individual budget has radically changed Jonathan's life in several ways:

*   He is happier. He is doing things he enjoys and is learning more quickly than he ever has done.
*   He is contributing, working, doing deliveries and meeting different people.
*   He is much more active, getting out in the fresh air which he enjoys and which keeps him fitter.

All of this has resulted in significant efficiency savings in the costs of Jonathan's care: over £100,000 in hospital stays, over £300,000 in residential care costs and over £100,000 in education funding.

Source: Alakeson and Duffy (2011)

References

ADASS (Association of Directors of Adult Social Services) (2012) *Personal budgets survey March 2012* (www.adass.org.uk/images/stories/Policy%20Networks/Resources/Key%20Documents/PersonalBudgetsSurveyMarch2012.pdf).

ADASS and the South West Regional Improvement and Efficiency Partnership (2010) *The self-directed support process – What does 'good' look like?*, London: Think Local Act Personal.

Alakeson, V. (2010) *International developments in self-directed care*, New York: Commonwealth Fund.

Alakeson, V. (2012) *Personal health budgets for continuing healthcare: 10 features of an effective process*, Wythall: In Control and Transition Alliance.

Alakeson, V. and Duffy, S. (2011) *Health efficiencies: The possible impact of personalisation in healthcare*, Sheffield: Centre for Welfare Reform.

Alakeson, V. and Perkins, R. (2012) *Recovery, personalisation and personal budgets*, London: Centre for Mental Health.

Alakeson, V. and Rosen, R. (2011) 'Chronic disease and integrated care', in J. Smith and K. Walsche (eds) *Healthcare management*, London: McGraw Hill International, pp 188–213.

Alakeson, V., Miller, C. and Bunin, A. (2013) *Coproduction of health and wellbeing outcomes: The new paradigm for effective health and social care*, London: Office for Public Management.

Arnold, C. (2010) *Bedlam: London and its mad*, London: Pocket Books.

Arntz, M. and Thomsen, S. (2008a) *Reforming home care provision in Germany: Evidence from a social experiment*, ZEW Discussion Papers 08-114, Mannheim: Centre for European Economic Research.

Arntz, M. and Thomsen, S. (2008b) *Crowding out informal care? Evidence from a social experiment in Germany*, ZEW Discussion Papers 08-113, Mannheim: Centre for European Economic Research.

Arthritis Research UK (2012) *Personal health budgets: Perspectives from people with arthritis and other musculoskeletal conditions*, London: Arthritis Research UK.

Audit Commission (2012) *Making personal health budgets financially sustainable: Practical suggestions on how to manage financial risk*, London: Audit Commission.

Bennett, H.D., Coleman, E.A., Parry, C., Bodenheimer, T. and Chen, E.H. (2010) 'Health coaching for patients with chronic illness', *Family Practice Management* (http://selfmanagementsupport.health.org.uk/media_manager/public/179/SMS_resource-centre_publications/Bodenheimer%20HealthCoachArticle.pdf).

Bennett, S. (2012) *Personal health budgets guide: Implications for NHS-funded providers*, London: Department of Health.

Bennett, S. and Stockton, S. (2011) *Best practice in direct payments support – A guide for commissioners*, London: Joint Improvement Partnership and Groundswell.

Bennett, S. and Stockton, S. (2012) *Personal health budgets guide: Integrating personal budgets – early learning*, London: Department of Health.

Beresford, P. (2012) 'Are personal budgets really the way ahead for social care?', *The Guardian online*, 17 January (wwww.guardian.co.uk/social-care-network/2012/jan/17/personal-budgets-way-ahead-social).

Berwick, D. (2009a) 'What patient-centered care really means' (www.youtube.com/watch?v=SSauhroFTpk).

Berwick, D. (2009b) 'What "patient-centered" should mean: Confessions of an extremist', *Health Affairs*, vol 28, no 4, w555–w565.

BMA (British Medical Association) (2012) 'Government set to push ahead with personal health budgets', 2 November (http://bma.org.uk/news-views-analysis/news/2012/november/government-set-to-push-ahead-with-personal-health-budgets).

Boyle, D., Coote, A., Sherwood, C. and Slay, J. (2010) *Right here right now. Taking co-production into the mainstream*, London: New Economics Foundation and Nesta.

Brewis, R. and Fitzgerald, J. (2012) 'Personal health budgets in practice: the experience of individuals and families', Presentation given at 'Independence pays: What do personal health budgets mean for the NHS?', Health Services Management Centre, University of Birmingham, 11 October.

Brewis, R., Stewart, G. and Fitzgerald, J. (2012) *Personal health budgets guide: Implementing effective care planning*, London: Department of Health.

Brindle, D. (2010) 'Boost for cost effective individual budgets', *The Guardian*, 28 January.

Brown, R., Carlson, B.L., Dale, S., Foster, L., Phillips, B. and Schore, J. (2007) *Cash & Counseling: Improving the lives of Medicaid beneficiaries who need personal care or home- and community-based services. Final report*, Princeton, NJ: Mathematica Policy Research, Inc.

Campbell, N., Cockerell, R., Porter, S., Strong, S., Ward, L. and Williams, V. (2011) *Independent living strategy: Support planning and brokerage. Final report from the support planning and brokerage demonstration project*, London: Office for Disability Issues.

Carr, S. (2010) *Enabling risk, ensuring safety: Self-directed support and personal budgets*, London: Social Care Institute for Excellence.

Cattermole, M. (2012a) *Personal health budgets guide: Budget setting for NHS continuing healthcare*, London: Department of Health.

Cattermole, M. (2012b) *Personal health budgets guide: How to set budgets – Early learning from the personal health budget pilot*, London: Department of Health.

Cattermole, M. (2012c) *Personal health budgets guide. How to get good results. Key learning from the evaluation*, London: Department of Health.

Cattermole, M. (2012d) *Personal health budgets guide: Market development case study: Dorset*, London: Department of Health.

Cesar, V., Habicht, J.-P. and Bryce, J. (2004) 'Evidence-based public health: Moving beyond randomized trials', *American Journal of Public Health*, vol 94, no 3, pp 400-5.

Colhoun, A. and Porter, S. (2012) 'Substance misuse personalisation. Croydon's work to date – overview and reflections', Presentation given at Royal College of Psychiatrists seminar, 5 October (www.rcpsych.ac.uk/pdf/rcpsych%20croydondaat%20for%20circulation.pdf).

Cook, J., Russell, C., Grey, D. and Jonikas, J. (2008) 'Economic grand rounds: a self-directed care model for mental health recovery', *Psychiatric Services*, vol 59, no 6, pp 600-2.

Coulter, A. and Collins, A. (2011) *Making shared decision-making a reality: No decision about me, without me*, London: The King's Fund.

Coyle, D. (2009) *Recovery budgets in a mental health service. Evaluating recovery budgets for people accessing an early intervention service and the impact of working with self-directed services on the team members within a North West of England NHS Trust*, Liverpool: Merseycare NHS Trust.

CQC (Care Quality Commission) (2011) *Dignity and nutrition inspection programme: National overview*, Newcastle: CQC.

Craston, M., Thom, G., Johnson, R. and Henderson, L. (2012) *Evaluation of the SEND pathfinder programme: Interim evaluation report*, London: Department for Education.

Crisp, N. (2010) *Turning the world upside down: The search for global health in the 21st century*, London: Royal Society of Medicine Press.

Cummins, J. and Miller, C. (2007) *Coproduction and social capital: The role that users and citizens play in improving local services*, London: Office for Public Management.

Dale, S. and Brown, R. (2006) 'Reducing nursing home use through consumer directed personal care services', *Medical Care*, vol 44, no 8, pp 760-7.

Dale, S., Brown, R. and Philips, B. (2004) *Does Arkansas' Cash & Counseling affect service use and public costs?*, Princeton, NJ: Mathematica Policy Research Inc.

Davidson, J., Baxter, K., Glendinning, C., Jones, K., Forder, J., Caiels, J., Welch, E., Windle, K., Dolan, P. and King, D. (2012) *Personal health budgets: Experiences and outcomes for budget holders at nine months. Fifth interim report*, London: Department of Health.

Deegan, P. (2005) 'The importance of personal medicine: A qualitative study of resilience in people with psychiatric disabilities', *Scandinavian Journal of Public Health*, vol 33, no 66, pp 29–35.

Deegan, P. (2008) 'Recovery from mental disorders: A lecture' (www.youtube.com/watch?v=jhK-7DkWaKE).

Deegan, P. and Drake, R. (2006) 'Shared decision-making and medication management in the recovery process', *Psychiatric Services Journal*, vol 57, no 11, pp 1636–9.

Devon Partnership NHS Trust (2011) *Quality account 2010/11*, Exeter: Devon Partnership NHS Trust.

DfE (Department for Education) (2011) *Support and aspiration: A new approach to special educational needs and disability* – London: DfE.

DH (Department of Health) (1999) *National Service Framework for mental health: Modern standards and service models*, London: DH.

DH (2005) *MORI survey: Public attitudes to self-care baseline survey*, London: DH.

DH (2008) *High quality care for all*, London: DH.

DH (2010a) *Direct payments for healthcare: Information for pilot sites*, London: DH.

DH (2010b) *A vision for adult social care: Capable communities and active citizens*, London: DH.

DH (2011a) *A simple guide to Payment by Results*, London: DH.

DH (2011b) *Martin's story from the personal health budget pilot* (www.personalhealthbudgets.england.nhs.uk/Topics/latest/Resource/index.cfm?cid=8330&excludepageid=0).

DH (2011c) *The operating framework for the NHS in England 2012/13*, London: DH.

DH (2012a) *Transforming care: A national response to Winterbourne View Hospital. A Department of Health review: Final report*, London: DH.

DH (2012b) *The mandate. A mandate from the government to the NHS Commissioning Board: April 2013 to March 2015*, London: DH.

DH (2012c) 'Personal health budgets to be rolled out', 30 November (www.dh.gov.uk/health/2012/11/phb).

DH (2012e) 'Introduction to personal health budgets' (www.personalhealthbudgets.dh.gov.uk/Topics/Toolkit/Intro).

DH (2012f) *Draft mental health Payment by Results guidance for 2013-14*, London: DH.

DH (2012g) *Overview of Health and Social Care Act fact sheet* (https://www.gov.uk/government/uploads/system/uploads/attachment_data/file/138257/A1.-Factsheet-Overview-240412.pdf).

DH (2012h) *Tom's story* (www.personalhealthbudgets.dh.gov.uk/_library/Resources/Personalhealthbudgets/2012/TomsStory.pdf).

DH (2013) *Direct payments for healthcare. A consultation on updated policy for regulations*, London: DH.

Dixon, A. and Ashton, B. (2008) 'Super patients should use their powers wisely' (www.kingsfund.org.uk/publications/articles/super-patients-should-use-their-powers-wisely).

Dixon, A., Appleby, J., Robertson, R., Burge, P., Devlin, N. and Magee, H. (2010) *Patient choice: How patients choose and providers respond*, London: The King's Fund.

Doty, P. and O'Keeffe, J. (2010) 'Self-direction and healthcare', in J. O'Keeffe (ed) *Developing and implementing self-direction programs and policies*, Boston, MA: National Resource Center for Participant-directed Services, pp 9-1–9-24.

Dowson, S. (2007) *Ten statements about support brokers*, National Support Broker Network (www.nationalbrokeragenetwork.org.uk/wp-content/uploads/2012/11/10_statements_about_support_brokers.pdf).

DRC (Disability Rights Commission) (2002) *Policy statement on social care and independent living*, London: DRC.

Duffy, S. (2011a) *A fair society and the limits of personalisation*, Sheffield: Centre for Welfare Reform.

Duffy, S. (2011b) *Simplify the RAS* (www.centreforwelfarereform.org/library/type/text/simplify-the-ras.html).

Duffy, S. and Fulton, K. (2009) *Should we ban brokerage?*, Sheffield: Centre for Welfare Reform.

Edwards, A. and Elwyn, G. (2009) 'Shared decision making in healthcare: achieving evidence-based patient choice', in A. Edwards and E. Elwyn (eds) *Shared decision making in healthcare: Achieving evidence-based patient choice* (2nd edn), Oxford: Oxford University Press, pp 3-10.

Eost-Telling, C. (2010) *Stockport self-directed support pilot in mental health. Final report of the evaluation of the self-directed support pilot*, Chester: University of Chester.

Epstein, R.M., Fiscella, K., Lesser, C.S. and Stange, K.C. (2010) 'Why the nation needs a policy push on patient-centered health care', *Health Affairs*, vol 29, no 8, pp 1489-95.

Evans, J. (2003) *The Independent Living Movement in the UK* (www.independentliving.org/docs6/evans2003.html).

Exley, C., Bamford, C. and Hughes, J. (2011) *Advance care planning: An opportunity for person-centred care for people living with dementia*, Newcastle: Institute of Health and Society, Newcastle University.

Fitzgerald, J., Murray-Neill, R. and Simpson, B. (2012a) *Personal health budgets guide: Ways in which the money can be held and managed*, London: Department of Health.

Fitzgerald, J., Brewis, R., Macintyre, L., Royle, C. and Tyson, A. (2012b) *Personal health budgets guide: Third party organisations: The families' perspective*, London: Department of Health.

Florida Department of Children and Families (2007) *Report on the effectiveness of the Self-directed Care Community Mental Health Treatment Program as required by s.394.9084 FS*, Tallahassee, FL: Mental Health Program Office, Florida Department of Children and Families.

Forder, J., Jones, K., Glendinning, C., Caiels, J., Welch, W., Baxter, K., Davidson, J., Windle, K., Irvine, A., King, D. and Dolan, P. (2012) *Evaluation of the personal health budget pilot programme*, London: Department of Health.

Fox, A. (2012) *Personalisation: Lessons from social care*, London: RSA Action and Research Centre.

Francis, R. (2013) *Report of the Mid Staffordshire NHS Foundation Trust Public Inquiry*, London: The Stationery Office.

Gadsby, E. (2013) *Personal budgets and health: A review of the evidence*, London: Policy Research Unit in Commissioning and the Healthcare System.

Gibson, P.G., Powell, H., Wilson, A., Abramson, M.J., Haywood, P., Bauman, A., Hensley, M.J., Walters, E.H. and Roberts, J.J.L. (2004) 'Self-management education and regular practitioner review for adults with asthma', *The Cochrane Library*, Issue 2, Chichester: John Wiley & Sons.

Glasby, J. (2008) *Individual budgets and the interface with health: A discussion paper for the Care Services Improvement Partnership (CSIP)*, Birmingham: Health Services Management Centre.

Glasby, J. (2011a) *Evidence, policy and practice: Critical perspectives in health and social care*, Bristol: The Policy Press.

Glasby, J. (2011b) *Whose risk is it anyway? Risk and regulation in an era of personalisation*, York: Joseph Rowntree Foundation.

Glasby, J. (2012) *Commissioning for health and well-being: An introduction*, Bristol: The Policy Press.

Glasby, J. and Hasler, F. (2004) *A healthy option? Direct payments and the implications for health care*, Birmingham: Health Services Management Centre/London: National Centre for Independent Living.

Glasby, J. and Littlechild, R. (2002) *Social work and direct payments*, Bristol: The Policy Press.

Glasby, J. and Littlechild, R. (2009) *Direct payments and personal budgets: Putting personalisation into practice* (2nd edn), Bristol: The Policy Press.

Glasby, J., Walshe, K. and Harvey, G. (eds) (2007) 'Evidence-based practice', *Special edition of Evidence & Policy*, vol 3, no 3, pp 323-457.

Glasby, J., Ham, C., Littlechild, R. and McKay, S. (2010) *The case for social care reform – The wider economic and social benefits. Final report*, Birmingham: University of Birmingham.

Glendinning, C., Halliwell, S., Jacobs, S., Rummery, K. and Tyrer, J. (2000a) 'Bridging the gap: Using direct payments to purchase integrated care', *Health and Social Care in the Community*, vol 8, no 3, pp 192-200.

Glendinning, C., Halliwell, S., Jacobs, S., Rummery, K. and Tyrer, J. (2000b) *Buying independence: Using direct payments to integrate health and social services*, Bristol: The Policy Press.

Glendinning, C., Challis, D., Fernandez, J., Jacobs, S., Jones, K., Knapp, M., Manthorpe, J., Moran, N., Netten, A., Stevens, M. and Wilberforce, M. (2008) *Evaluation of the Individual Budgets Pilot Programme. Final report*, York: University of York.

Gordon, C., Leigh, J., Kay, D., Humphries, S., Tee, K.-S., Winch, J. and Thorne, W. (2012) *Evaluation of the consumer-directed care initiative: Final report*, Canberra: KPMG.

Hannan, A. (2010) 'Real-time digital medicine', Presentation given at the International Quality Improvement Exchange, Cameron House Hotel, Loch Lomond, 4-6 March.

Hasnain-Wynia, R. (2006) 'Is evidence-based medicine patient-centered and is patient-centered care evidence-based?', *Health Services Research*, vol 41, no 1, pp 1-8.

Hatton, C. and Waters, J. (2011) *The national personal budget survey*, London: Think Local Act Personal.

Health Foundation (2010) *Personal health budgets: Research scan*, London: Health Foundation.

Hibbard, J.H., Stockard, J., Mahoney, E.R. and Tusler, M. (2004) 'Development of the Patient Activation Measure (PAM): Conceptualising and measuring activation in patients and consumers', *Health Services Research*, vol 39, no 4, pt 1, pp 1005-26.

HM Government (2007) *Putting People First: A shared vision and commitment to the transformation of adult social care*, London: HM Government.

HM Government (2011) *Open public services*, White Paper, London: Cabinet Office.

HM Treasury and DfES (Department for Education and Skills) (2005) *Support for parents: The best start for children*, London: The Stationery Office.

Holder, H. and Thorlby, R. (2012) *The new NHS in England: Structure and accountabilities*, London: The Nuffield Trust.

Horne, M., Khan, H. and Corrigan, P. (2013) *People-powered Health: Health for people, by people and with people*, London: Nesta and Innovation Unit.

Hough, J. and Rice, B. (2010) *Providing personalised support to rough sleepers*, York: Joseph Rowntree Foundation.

House of Commons Health Committee (2005) *NHS continuing healthcare. Sixth report of session 2004-5*, London: The Stationery Office Ltd.

Humphries, R. and Curry, N. (2011) *Integrating health and social care: Where next?*, London: The King's Fund.

Imison, C. (2011) *Transforming our healthcare system: Ten priorities for commissioners*, London: The King's Fund.

Innovation Unit (2012a) *Working towards people-powered health: Insights from practitioners*, London: Nesta.

Innovation Unit (2012b) *People-powered health: Project summaries*, London: Nesta.

Institute of Medicine (2001) *Crossing the quality chasm*, Washington, DC: National Academies Press.

Irvine, A., Davidson, J., Glendinning, C., Jones, K., Forder, J., Caiels, J., Welch, E., Windle, K., Dolan, P. and King, D. (2011) *Personal health budgets: Early experiences of budget holders*, London: Department of Health.

Jones, K., Forder, J., Caiels, J., Welch, E., Windle, K., Davidson, J., Dolan, P., Glendinning, C., Irvine, A. and King, D. (2011) *The cost of implementing personal health budgets*, PSSRU Discussion Paper, London: Department of Health.

Jones, R. (2012) *Personalisation and social care* (www.nuffieldtrust.org.uk/talks/videos/richard-jones-personalisation-and-social-care).

Kelly, E. and Tetlow, G. (2012) *Choosing the place of care: The effect of patient choice on treatment location in England, 2003-2011*, London: The Nuffield Trust and Institute for Fiscal Studies.

Lansley, A. (2012) *The National Health Service and public health service in England: Secretary of State's annual report 2011/2012*, London: HM Government.

Leadbeater, C. (2004) *Personalisation through participation. A new script for public services*, London: Demos.

Le Grand, J. (2007) *The other invisible hand: Delivering public services through choice and competition*, Princeton, NJ: Princeton University Press.

Lewis, S. (2011) 'Personal budgets policy could lead to "top ups", RCN warns', *Nursing Times*, 10 October.

Lorig, K., Sobel, D. and Stewart, A. (1999) 'Evidence suggesting that a chronic disease self-management program can improve health status while reducing utilization and costs: A randomized trial', *Medical Care*, vol 37, no 1, pp 5-14.

Marsh, C. and Fox, C. (2012) 'Could personalisation reduce offending', Presentation given at Academy Justice Commissioning Seminar, 15 November.

Mathers, N., Thomas, M. and Patel, V. (2012) *Personal health budgets: RCGP position statement*, London: Royal College of General Practitioners.

Maule, E. (2010) 'CRIF: Self-directed Care, Delaware County, PA', Presentation to the Office of Mental Health and Substance Abuse Services (OMHSAS) Joint Advisory Committee, 4 March.

Mencap (2009) 'Institutional hospitals a thing of the past' (www.mencap.org.uk/node/7173).

Milburn, A. (2007) 'A 2020 vision for public services', Speech at the London School of Economics and Political Science, 16 May.

Miller, R., Dickinson, H. and Glasby, J. (2011) 'The care trust pilgrims', *Journal of Integrated Care*, vol 19, no 4, pp 14-21.

Moreton, C. (2012) 'Baroness Campbell: "Disabled people are the best problem solvers"', *Daily Telegraph*, 8 December.

Morris, J. (1993) *Independent lives: Community care and disabled people*, London: Macmillan.

Mulgan, G. (2012) 'Government with the people: the outlines of the relational state', in G. Cooke and R. Muir (eds) *The relational state: How recognising the importance of human relationships could revolutionise the role of the state*, London: Institute for Public Policy Research, pp 20-34.

Murphy, M.G., Selkow, I., Crisp, S. and Mahoney, K.J. (2012) *Agency with choice: Key components for practical implementation while maintaining participant choice and control*, Boston, MA: National Resource Center for Participant-Directed Services.

Murray, P. and Duffy, S. (2011) *Real wealth*, Sheffield: The Centre for Welfare Reform (www.centreforwelfarereform.org/library/by-date/real-wealth.html).

National Audit Office (2011) *Oversight of user choice and provider competition in care markets*, London: National Audit Office.

National Collaborating Centre for Mental Health (2010) *Depression in adults with a chronic physical health problem: Treatment and management*, London: British Psychological Society and Royal College of Psychiatrists.

Naylor, C. (2012) *PCTs and CCGs – Not so different after all* (www.kingsfund.org.uk/blog/2012/07/ccgs-and-pcts-not-so-different-after-all).

NCIL (National Centre for Independent Living) (2008) *The Direct Payments Development Fund* (www.ncil.org.uk/imageuploads/file/DHreport2.pdf).

Needham, C. (2011) *Personalising public services: Understanding the personalisation narrative*, Bristol: The Policy Press.

Needham, C. (2012) *What is happening to day centre services? Voices from frontline staff*, Birmingham: University of Birmingham and Unison.

Nene CCG (Clinical Commissioning Group) (2012) *Personal health budgets* (www.neneccg.nhs.uk/personal-health-budgets).

Newman S., Steed, L. and Mulligan, K. (2004) 'Self-management interventions for chronic illness', *Lancet*, vol 364, pp 1523-37.

NHS Commissioning Board (2012) *Everyone counts: Planning for patients 2013/14*, London: NHS.

NHS Confederation (2012) *Joint personal budgets: A new solution to the problem of integrated care?*, London: NHS Confederation and Association of Directors of Adult Social Services.

NMHDU (National Mental Health Development Unit) (2010) *Examples of peer support initiatives* (www.nmhdu.org.uk/silo/files/peer-support-initiatives-word-doc.do).

NMHDU (2011a) *Facing up to the challenge of personal health budgets: The view of frontline professionals*, London: NHS Confederation.

NMHDU (2011b) *Personal health budgets: The views of service users and carers*, London: NHS Confederation.

Norris, W., Warnick, T., Moreno, L., Warren, J. and Razzano, L. (2010) 'Self-directing your own recovery by controlling you own service dollars', Presentation given at 'Alternatives 2010 – Promoting wellness through social justice', Anaheim, CA, 1 October.

O'Hagan, M. (1993) *Stopovers on my way home from Mars*, London: Survivors Speak Out.

OPPAGA (Office of Program Policy Analysis and Government Accountability) (2010) *Insufficient information available to fully assess the success of the Self-directed Care program*, Report No 10-40, Tallahassee, FL: OPPAGA.

Policy and International Department (2011) *Personal health budgets: An overview of policy in England so far*, London: Royal College of Nursing.

Ramesh, R. (2012) 'Hundreds of contracts signed in "biggest ever act of NHS privatization"', *The Guardian*, 3 October.

RCP (Royal College of Psychiatrists) (2012) *National audit of schizophrenia 2012*, London: Health Quality Improvement Partnership and RCP.

Reeves, R. (2010) *A Liberal dose? Health and well being – the role of the state. An independent report* (http://base-uk.org/sites/base-uk.org/files/[user-raw]/11-06/rr.pdf).

Repper, J. and Carter, T. (2010) 'A review of the literature on peer support in mental health services', *Journal of Mental Health*, vol 20, no 4, pp 392-411.

Repper, J. and Perkins, R. (2003) *Social inclusion and recovery: A model for mental health practice*, London: Baillière Tindall.

Reynolds, T. (2012) 'Personal health budgets in practice: the example of continuing health care', Presentation given at 'Independence pays: What do personal health budgets mean for the NHS?', Birmingham: Health Services Management Centre, University of Birmingham, 11 October.

Richards, N. and Coulter, A. (2007) *Is the NHS becoming more patient-centred? Trends from the national surveys of NHS patients 2002–7*, Oxford: Picker Institute Europe.

Roberts, A., Marshall, L. and Charlesworth, A. (2012) *A decade of austerity?*, London: Nuffield Trust.

Rogers, A., Bower, P., Gardner, C., Gately, C., Kennedy, A., Lee, V., Middleton, E., Reeves, D. and Richardson, G. (2006) *The national evaluation of the pilot phase of the Expert Patient Programme. Final report*, Manchester: National Primary Care Research & Development Centre, University of Manchester.

Routledge, M. and Lewis, J. (2011) *Taking stock, moving forward*, London: Think Local Act Personal.

RWJF (Robert Wood Johnson Foundation) (2006) *Choosing independence: An overview of the Cash & Counseling model of self-directed personal assistance services*, Princeton, NJ: RWJF.

Samuel, M. (2012) 'Expert guide to direct payments, personal budgets and individual budgets', *Community Care*, 25 July.

SCIE (Social Care Institute for Excellence) and nef (New Economics Foundation) (2011) *Budgets and beyond: Interim report*, London: SCIE and nef.

Secretary of State for Health (2012) *Draft Care and Support Bill*, London: The Stationery Office.

Sen, A. (1999) *Development as freedom*, Oxford: Oxford University Press.

Sen, A. (2010) *The idea of justice*, London: Penguin.

Singh, D. and Ham, C. (2006) *Improving care for people with long-term conditions: A review of UK and international frameworks*, Birmingham: Health Services Management Centre and NHS Institute for Innovation and Improvement.

Slade, E. (2012) *Feasibility of expanding self-directed services to people with serious mental illness*, Washington, DC: Office of the Assistant Secretary for Planning and Evaluation.

Stevens, L. (2011) *Creating the conditions for co-production within an outcomes approach to commissioning in Camden*, London: New Economics Foundation.

Steventon, A. (2012) 'How useful are randomised controlled trials in evaluating new ways of delivering care?', London: Nuffield Trust (www.nuffieldtrust.org.uk/blog/how-useful-are-randomised-controlled-trials-evaluating-new-ways-delivering-health-care).

Sullivan, A. (2006) *Empowerment initiatives brokerage: Service quality and outcome evaluation*, Portland, OR: Oregon Technical Assistance Corporation.

Tarr, A. (2011) *Personalising welfare to work: The case for personal welfare budgets*, London: Inclusion.

Tu, T.U., Lambert, C., Navin Shah, J., Westwood, P. (2012) *Right to Control Trailblazers process evaluation: Wave 1*, London: Office for Disability Issues.

Tyson, A., Brewis, R., Crosby, N., Hatton, C., Stansfield, J., Tomlinson, C., Waters, J. and Wood, A. (2010) *A report on In Control's third phase. Evaluation and learning 2008-2009*, London: In Control Publications.

Unison (2009) *Unison briefing: Personal health budgets in the NHS* (www.unison.org.uk/file/A8909.pdf).

Wagner, E. (1998) 'Chronic disease management: what will it take to improve care for chronic illness?', *Effective Clinical Practice*, vol 1, pp 2-4.

Wallace, L.M., Turner, A., Kosmala-Anderson, J., Sharma, S,. Jesuthasan, J., Bourne, C. and Realpe, A. (2012) *Co-creating Health: Evaluation of first phase*, London: Health Foundation.

Walton, G. (2012) 'Clinical commissioning versus individual commissioning: The role of personal health budgets', Presentation given at Nuffield Trust Seminar, 26 April.

White, C. (2011) *The personal touch: The Dutch experience of personal health budgets*, London: Health Foundation.

WHO (World Health Organization) (2003) *Adherence to long-term therapies: Evidence for action*, Geneva: WHO.

Wilson, T. (2005) 'Rising to the challenge: will the NHS support people with long term conditions?', *British Medical Journal*, vol 330, pp 657-61.

Year of Care (2011) *Report of findings from the pilot programme,* London: Health Foundation, Department of Health, Diabetes UK and NHS Diabetes.

Zarb, G. and Nadash, P. (1994) *Cashing in on independence: Comparing the costs and benefits of cash and services,* London: British Council of Disabled People.

Index

Note: The following abbreviations have been used – *f* = figure; *t* = table.